Auditory Impairment and Assistive Hearing SOURCEBOOK

SECOND EDITION

Disability Series

Auditory Impairment and Assistive Hearing SOURCEBOOK

SECOND EDITION

Basic Consumer Health Information about Auditory Health, Types of Auditory Impairment, Conditions Leading to Hearing Loss, and Assistive Hearing Devices for Improving the Quality of Life for Individuals with Hearing Impairment

Along with Information on Disability Rights, Employment Protections, Communication Tools, and Resources for Additional Help and Support

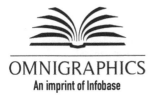

OMNIGRAPHICS
An imprint of Infobase

Bibliographic Note
Because this page cannot legibly accommodate all the copyright notices,
the Bibliographic Note portion of the Preface constitutes an extension
of the copyright notice.

* * *

OMNIGRAPHICS
An imprint of Infobase
8 The Green
Suite #19225
Dover, DE 19901
www.infobase.com
James Chambers, *Editorial Director*

* * *

Copyright © 2025 Infobase
ISBN 978-0-7808-2164-4
E-ISBN 978-0-7808-2165-1

Library of Congress Cataloging-in-Publication Data

Title: Auditory impairment and assistive hearing sourcebook / edited by James Chambers.

Description: Second edition. | Dover, DE: Omnigraphics, an imprint of Infobase, [2025] | Series: Disability series | Includes index. | Summary: Provides essential health information about auditory impairment, including its types, causes, and related disorders such as genetic, age-related, and infection-based hearing loss, along with guidance on diagnosis, treatment, prevention, assistive hearing technologies, and disability rights. Includes an index and resources for additional information-- Provided by publisher.

Identifiers: LCCN 2024045632 (print) | LCCN 2024045633 (ebook) | ISBN 9780780821644 | ISBN 9780780821651 eISBN

Subjects: LCSH: Self-help devices for people with disabilities | Hard of hearing people--Rehabilitation | LCGFT: Handbooks and manuals

Classification: LCC RF297 .A93 2024 (print) | LCC RF297 (ebook) | DDC 362.4/2--dc23/eng

LC record available at https://lccn.loc.gov/2024045632

LC ebook record available at https://lccn.loc.gov/2024045633

Electronic or mechanical reproduction, including photography, recording, or any other information storage and retrieval system for the purpose of resale is strictly prohibited without permission in writing from the publisher.

The information in this publication was compiled from the sources cited and from other sources considered reliable. While every possible effort has been made to ensure reliability, the publisher will not assume liability for damages caused by inaccuracies in the data, and makes no warranty, express or implied, on the accuracy of the information contained herein.

This book is printed on acid-free paper meeting the ANSI Z39.48 Standard. The infinity symbol that appears above indicates that the paper in this book meets that standard.

Printed in the United States

Table of Contents

Preface | ix

Part 1: Introduction to Auditory Impairment
Chapter 1——The Fundamentals of Sound and the Auditory System | 3
Chapter 2——Understanding Hearing Loss | 9
    Section 2.1——Overview of Hearing Loss | 10
    Section 2.2——Hearing Loss in Infants and Children | 12
    Section 2.3——Hearing Loss in Older Adults | 16
Chapter 3——Auditory Impairment and Quality of Life | 23
    Section 3.1——Effects of Hearing Loss on Daily Life and Well-Being | 24
    Section 3.2——Barriers to Accessibility and Participation | 26
    Section 3.3——Addressing Communication Needs in Auditory Impairment | 30
Chapter 4——Communicating with People with Hearing Loss | 35
    Section 4.1——American Sign Language | 36
    Section 4.2——Telecommunications Relay Service | 38

Part 2: Effect of Noise on Hearing Loss
Chapter 5——Noise-Induced Hearing Loss | 45
Chapter 6——Workplace Noise | 49
    Section 6.1——Effects of Workplace Noise on Hearing Health | 50
    Section 6.2——Occupational Noise Risks in Music and Aviation | 51
    Section 6.3——Hearing Loss in the Forestry and Logging Industry | 53
    Section 6.4——Effective Noise Reduction Techniques in the Workplace | 56

Part 3: Auditory Impairment: Diseases and Related Disorders

Chapter 7—Infectious Diseases and Hearing Loss | 63
    Section 7.1—Ear Infections in Children | 64
    Section 7.2—Meningitis | 67
    Section 7.3—Shingles | 73

Chapter 8—Congenital and Developmental Hearing Loss | 79
    Section 8.1—Congenital Cytomegalovirus and Its Effect on Hearing | 80
    Section 8.2—Enlarged Vestibular Aqueducts and Hearing Loss | 82

Chapter 9—Chronic and Acquired Disorders | 87
    Section 9.1—Ménière Disease | 88
    Section 9.2—Tinnitus | 90
    Section 9.3—Otosclerosis | 96
    Section 9.4—Balance Disorders | 97
    Section 9.5—Auditory Neuropathy | 103
    Section 9.6—Sudden Deafness | 106
    Section 9.7—Hearing Problems as a Late Effect of Childhood Cancer Treatment | 109
    Section 9.8—Congenital Zika Syndrome | 111

Chapter 10—Age-Related Hearing Loss | 115

Chapter 11—Genetic Factors in Hearing Loss | 119

Part 4: Diagnosis, Prevention, and Treatment for Auditory Impairment

Chapter 12—Diagnosis of Hearing Loss | 127
    Section 12.1—Newborn Hearing Screening | 128
    Section 12.2—Hearing Tests for Adults | 130

Chapter 13—Preventing Noise-Induced Auditory Loss | 135
    Section 13.1—Protecting Your Hearing from Noise-Induced Damage | 136
    Section 13.2—Selecting and Using Effective Hearing Protectors | 138
    Section 13.3—Strategies for Preventing Noise-Induced Hearing Loss in Students | 140
    Section 13.4—Strategies for Teaching Children to Protect Their Hearing | 143

Chapter 14—Intervention and Treatment for Auditory Impairment | 147
    Section 14.1—Intervention Strategies for Children with Hearing Loss | 148
    Section 14.2—Medications and Surgery for Hearing Loss in Children | 152
    Section 14.3—Steroid Treatments for Sudden Deafness | 153
    Section 14.4—Gene Therapy for Hearing Loss | 155

Part 5: Assistive Hearing for People with Auditory Impairment
Chapter 15—Hearing Aids | 161
Chapter 16—Over-the-Counter Hearing Aids | 167
Chapter 17—Cochlear Implants | 171
Chapter 18—Assistive Devices for Hearing Loss | 175
Chapter 19—Captioning and Visual Tools for Viewers with
    Hearing Impairments | 181

Part 6: Disability Rights for Auditory Impairment
Chapter 20—Legal Protections for People with Auditory
    Impairments | 189
Chapter 21—Hearing Impairments and Employment Rights | 195
Chapter 22—Support Structures for Auditory Impairment | 201
    Section 22.1—Supports in Hotels and Motels | 202
    Section 22.2—Supports in Hospital Settings | 204
Chapter 23—Service Animals: Rights and Responsibilities | 209
Chapter 24—Education | 215
    Section 24.1—Federal Requirements for Communication
        Access in Education | 216
    Section 24.2—Testing Accommodations and Disability
        Rights | 218

Part 7: Additional Resources
Chapter 25—Directory of Organizations Providing Support for People
    with Auditory Impairment | 225

Index | 233

Preface

ABOUT THIS BOOK

Auditory impairment can result from various factors, such as childhood illnesses, pregnancy-related complications, injury, hereditary conditions, age, or prolonged exposure to excessive noise. Hearing loss may range from mild to profound, with people facing different challenges depending on severity. Those with moderate impairment may struggle to distinguish speech patterns in conversation, while individuals with profound hearing loss may be unable to hear any sounds at all. According to the Centers for Disease Control and Prevention (CDC), in 2020, more than 98 percent of U.S. newborns were screened for hearing loss, and over 6,000 infants were identified with permanent hearing loss, yielding a prevalence rate of 1.8 per 1,000 babies screened. Hearing loss affects approximately 60.7 million Americans aged 12 and older, with about 44.1 million adults aged 20 and older experiencing some degree of hearing loss.

Auditory Impairment and Assistive Hearing Sourcebook, Second Edition begins with an overview of the auditory system and the effects of hearing loss on quality of life. The book details various types of hearing impairments, including those caused by genetic, congenital, infectious, and age-related factors. It discusses the effect of noise on hearing loss, including workplace noise and relevant regulations. It provides comprehensive information on diagnosing hearing loss, prevention strategies, and treatment options—such as medical and surgical interventions. It also explores assistive hearing technologies such as hearing aids, cochlear implants, and other devices, along with telecommunication services and accessibility support. The book concludes with resources for further help and information, including details on disability rights and services for people with hearing impairments.

HOW TO USE THIS BOOK

This book is divided into parts and chapters. Parts focus on broad areas of interest; chapters are devoted to single topics within a part.

Part 1: Introduction to Auditory Impairment provides a comprehensive overview of the auditory system and hearing loss, discussing various types of hearing loss across different age groups, such as infants, children, and older adults. It also explores the effects of auditory impairment on quality of life and effective communication methods for those with hearing loss.

Part 2: Effect of Noise on Hearing Loss examines noise-induced hearing loss, focusing on occupational noise exposure and its effects on hearing health. It discusses specific workplace settings, such as music, aviation, and forestry, and explores effective noise reduction techniques to safeguard hearing in these environments.

Part 3: Auditory Impairment: Diseases and Related Disorders addresses medical conditions that contribute to hearing loss, including infectious diseases (ear infections, meningitis), congenital conditions, chronic disorders (Ménière disease, tinnitus, otosclerosis), and age-related hearing loss. It also examines genetic factors influencing auditory impairment.

Part 4: Diagnosis, Prevention, and Treatment for Auditory Impairment focuses on diagnostic methods and preventive strategies for auditory impairment. It covers newborn screenings, hearing tests for adults, the prevention of noise-induced hearing loss, and treatment options, including medical interventions, surgical options, and emerging therapies such as gene therapy and steroid treatments for sudden deafness.

Part 5: Assistive Hearing for People with Auditory Impairment provides information on technologies and devices that assist people with hearing loss, including hearing aids, cochlear implants, and other assistive listening devices. It also discusses captioning and visual tools to aid communication for individuals with auditory impairments.

Part 6: Disability Rights for Auditory Impairment outlines the legal rights and protections for people with auditory impairments, including education and employment rights under the Americans with Disabilities Act (ADA). It discusses support systems in settings such as hotels, motels, and hospitals, and covers the role and rights of service animals.

Part 7: Additional Resources includes a directory of organizations and resources that provide information and support for individuals with auditory impairments.

BIBLIOGRAPHIC NOTE

This volume contains documents and excerpts from publications issued by the following U.S. government agencies: ADA.gov; Centers for Disease Control and Prevention (CDC); Federal Communications Commission (FCC); MedlinePlus; National Cancer Institute (NCI); National Center on Birth Defects and Developmental Disabilities (NCBDDD); National Institute for Occupational Safety and Health (NIOSH); National Institute of Neurological Disorders and Stroke (NINDS); National Institute on Aging (NIA); National Institute on Deafness and Other Communication Disorders (NIDCD); National Institutes of Health (NIH); Occupational Safety and Health Administration (OSHA); U.S. Department of Health and Human Services (HHS); and U.S. Equal Employment Opportunity Commission (EEOC).

ABOUT THE *DISABILITY SERIES*

At the request of librarians serving the one in four Americans living with a disability, as well as those seeking information to comprehend, navigate, and manage such conditions, the *Disability Series* was developed as a specialized collection within Omnigraphics' *Health Reference Series*. Each volume comprehensively addresses a specific topic chosen based on the needs and interests of these patrons. These volumes offer authoritative health information, serving as a reliable resource for librarians to equip consumers with the necessary facts to take charge of their well-being. This empowers individuals to better understand and address health challenges faced by themselves, family members, or loved ones. Patrons in search of this information can find answers in the *Disability Series*. The *Series*, however, is not designed for diagnosing disabilities, prescribing treatments, or substituting the health-care provider-patient relationship. Anyone concerned about medical symptoms, the potential for disability, or illness is encouraged to seek professional care from an appropriate health-care provider.

If you have suggestions for future *Disability Series* topics, please email us at: custserv@infobaselearning.com.

A NOTE ABOUT SPELLING AND STYLE

Disability Series editors use *Stedman's Medical Dictionary* as an authority for questions related to the spelling of medical terms and *The Chicago Manual of Style* for questions related to grammatical structures, punctuation, and other editorial concerns. Consistent adherence is not always possible, however, because the individual volumes within the *Series* include many documents from a wide variety of different producers, and the editor's primary goal is to present material from each source as accurately as is possible. This sometimes means that information in different chapters or sections may follow other guidelines and alternate spelling authorities. For example, occasionally a copyright holder may require that eponymous terms be shown in possessive forms (Crohn's disease vs. Crohn disease) or that British spelling norms be retained (leukaemia vs. leukemia).

Part 1 | Introduction to Auditory Impairment

Chapter 1 | The Fundamentals of Sound and the Auditory System

BASIC PRINCIPLES OF SOUND
Sound can be defined in the physical sense as a series of pressure waves caused by a vibrating object and propagated through an elastic medium. In other words, sound is initiated when an object begins to vibrate. As the object moves back and forth, it "bumps into" molecules in the surrounding area, forcing them to also move. These displaced molecules, in turn, put pressure on other molecules, thus propagating the sound wave. Because the molecules return to their original resting position following displacement, sound occurs in an "elastic" medium.

In the physiological sense, sound can be defined as the sensation evoked in the auditory system by these pressure changes.

Sound may be characterized along three main parameters:
- **Frequency**. It is the rate of the sound pressure waves, or how often the molecules are displaced in a given period. It is measured in Hertz (Hz), or cycles per second, and is perceived as pitch. Lower-pitched sounds (such as the rumble of traffic or a man's speaking voice) are lower in frequency; higher-pitched sounds (such as a whistle or a baby's cry) have higher frequencies.
- **Intensity**. It refers to the amplitude of the pressure waves, or how far the molecules are displaced from their original position. Amplitude is measured in decibels and is perceived as volume or loudness. Low-amplitude sounds (in which the molecules are displaced only a little) are

perceived as "quiet," and high-amplitude sounds (in which the displacements are larger) are perceived as "loud."
- **Complexity**. It refers to the interaction of the various frequencies and intensities that make up a sound. For example, a pure tone is a sound made up of only one frequency and one intensity. Pure tones do not exist in nature; most sounds comprise many frequencies at different intensities combined to create a complex signal. Complexity is perceived as sound quality or timbre. If a flute and violin are playing the same note at the same volume, complexity is the parameter of sound that allows us to distinguish between the two instruments.

HUMAN AUDITORY RANGE

Within the context of the National Health and Nutrition Examination Survey (NHANES), the primary focus will be on the frequency and intensity of signals. The human ear is responsive to frequencies from about 20 to 20,000 Hz but not equally so; it is most sensitive from about 1,000 to 3,000 Hz. The frequencies most necessary for understanding speech are 500–4,000 Hz, so the human ear is "tuned" to listen to human speech.

The human ear is responsive to a wide range of pressures. The pressure of a sound that is just barely audible to a young, normal-hearing listener is approximately 20 µPa (micropascal—a unit for measuring pressure). The pressure of a sound that is painfully loud could be as much as 200,000,000 µPa. Because it is cumbersome to use such a large range to quantify intensity, we use ratios to convert the pressure measurements to decibels. In decibels, the human ear is responsive to intensities from 0 to 140 dB—a much more manageable range.

BASIC PRINCIPLES OF AUDITION

When one thinks of the ear, they probably think primarily of the two most visible portions of the auditory system located on either side of the head. However, the ear consists of four main parts: the outer ear, the middle ear, the inner ear, and the auditory neural system (see Figure 1.1).

The Fundamentals of Sound and the Auditory System | 5

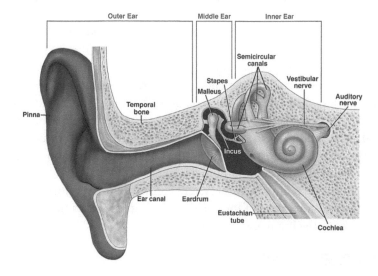

Figure 1.1. Ear
National Institute on Deafness and Other Communication Disorders (NIDCD)

The outer ear consists of the auricle (sometimes called the "pinna") and the ear canal (also called the "external auditory meatus"). It functions primarily to funnel sound into the ear and to modify the acoustic signal to some extent. The shape and size of the ear canal amplify signals with frequencies of approximately 2,000–3,000 Hz, which is the main reason that human hearing is most sensitive in this frequency range.

The middle ear consists of the eardrum (or tympanic membrane), three tiny bones (or ossicles) called the "malleus," "incus," and "stapes," and two small muscles. The primary function of the middle ear is to transform the acoustic signal into mechanical vibration. The middle ear muscles form part of a reflex arc (known as the "acoustic reflex"), which provides some protection against loud sounds. The middle ear also houses an opening to the eustachian tube, which connects this part of the ear to the back of the throat. The eustachian tube permits ventilation of the middle ear space, maintaining a balance in air pressure on either side of the eardrum; this balance is necessary for the eardrum to respond to sound most efficiently.

The inner ear consists of the cochlea, which is contained within a spiral opening in the temporal bone of the skull. The cochlea is divided into three parallel, fluid-filled ducts. The upper and lower ducts are connected at one end, and a wave is set up in them as the ossicles vibrate in response to sound. The middle duct contains rows of tiny hair cells. These hair cells bend as the wave reaches its peak; the bending of the hair cells stimulates the auditory nerve. The inner ear, therefore, transforms the mechanical vibrations from the middle ear into neural impulses.

Finally, the auditory neural system consists of the auditory nerve and the auditory areas of the cortex. This system carries the neural impulses to the brain and interprets them.

DEVELOPMENT OF AUDITORY FUNCTION

The auditory system is complete and possesses normal adult sensory function approximately halfway through prenatal development. However, the ability of the auditory neural system to process signals continues to develop for several years. Newborns can discriminate sounds based on frequency, intensity, and type of stimulus (they prefer human speech!). Over the first few months, infants learn to locate the source of sounds, associate hearing with their own vocal productions, and gradually improve their imitation of vocal sounds from others. By one year of age, they can process the meaning of approximately 50 words. By age four, children can process and understand just about everything they hear.

AGE-RELATED CHANGES IN HEARING

Auditory sensitivity reaches its peak during adolescence and then begins a gradual decline. Barring any insult that would accelerate this decline (such as noise or disease), the reduction in sensitivity is generally not clinically measurable until at least the third decade of life. After about age 60, hearing sensitivity decreases by an average of about 10 dB per decade. The decrease in hearing sensitivity begins at the highest frequencies and gradually progresses to include the middle and low frequencies. Hearing loss due to age-related changes is called "presbycusis."

There are several other age-related changes that occur in the ear. The cartilage in the outer ear and the ear canal begins to deteriorate, causing the auricle and canal opening to become very soft; this can lead to a condition known as "canal collapse," which can affect hearing test results. Additionally, the auricle enlarges, and the ear canal narrows, potentially shifting the resonant characteristics of the outer ear. Cerumen becomes drier, which—in combination with narrower ear canals—can impede the natural expulsion of wax from the ear. Cerumen may become more easily trapped, potentially partially or completely blocking the ear canal and causing a temporary loss of hearing. The tympanic membrane may become less flexible, and there can be slight degenerative changes in the joints between the bones in the middle ear. However, none of these issues are typically significant enough to affect hearing sensitivity.[1]

---

[1] "Audiometry Procedures," Centers for Disease Control and Prevention (CDC), December 2019. Available online. URL: wwwn.cdc.gov/nchs/data/nhanes/2019-2020/manuals/2019-Audiometry-Procedures-Manual-508.pdf. Accessed September 9, 2024.

Chapter 2 | Understanding Hearing Loss

Chapter Contents
Section 2.1—Overview of Hearing Loss...................................10
Section 2.2—Hearing Loss in Infants and Children........................12
Section 2.3—Hearing Loss in Older Adults...............................16

Section 2.1 | Overview of Hearing Loss

HEARING LOSS

Dysfunctions anywhere along the auditory pathway can cause hearing loss. Most hearing losses (such as age- and noise-related hearing losses) occur gradually over time, although sudden hearing losses (such as those resulting from infection or trauma) are also possible. Many sudden hearing losses are idiopathic, meaning the cause remains unknown. Hearing losses can be stable (not changing over time), progressive (worsening over time), or fluctuating (sometimes improving and sometimes worsening). Hearing losses may be categorized based on where in the ear the impairment is located (the type of hearing loss), how severely the impairment affects a person's hearing sensitivity (the degree of hearing loss), and which ears are affected (the laterality of the hearing loss).

TYPES OF HEARING LOSS

Hearing losses caused by a problem in the external or middle ear are referred to as "conductive hearing losses," because the difficulty lies in the conduction of sound to the cochlea. For example, excessive wax in the ear canal, fluid in the middle ear due to an infection, or a discontinuity between the ossicles can prevent sounds from efficiently reaching the inner ear. These types of hearing losses are often medically or surgically correctable.

Hearing losses caused by a problem in the inner ear or along the auditory nerve are known as "sensorineural hearing losses," because the difficulty lies in the ability of the cochlea to sense sound or the ability of the nerve to carry the signal to the brain. Damage to the cochlear hair cells due to age-related deterioration, repeated noise exposure, or a tumor on the auditory nerve are examples of etiologies leading to sensorineural hearing impairment. These types of hearing losses are not usually medically correctable. However, sensorineural hearing loss can often be remediated to a certain extent with hearing aids. While hearing aid technology has improved significantly in recent years, hearing aids do not restore normal hearing in the same way that eyeglasses restore normal vision.

A hearing loss can also be classified as mixed, meaning it is partly conductive and partly sensorineural. For example, if a person has a noise-induced hearing loss and then develops an ear infection, they would have a mixed hearing loss. The conductive portion of the hearing loss may resolve when the infection clears up, but the sensorineural portion is generally permanent.

CLASSIFYING THE DEGREE OF HEARING LOSS

Classifying the degree of hearing loss is more complex. The severity of the handicap due to abnormal hearing thresholds depends on several interrelated factors, such as the age of the individual, the age at which the impairment was first sustained, the location of the damage within the auditory system, the individual's communicative environment and needs, and the presence or absence of other illnesses or sensory deficits. For instance, a person who has experienced significant hearing loss since birth is affected differently than someone who acquires a similar hearing loss after reaching adulthood. A person with conductive hearing loss (which typically causes a reduction in the audibility of sounds) is affected differently than someone with sensorineural hearing loss (which often causes a reduction in both the intelligibility and audibility of sounds), even if their thresholds are the same. Furthermore, a person whose only sensory impairment is hearing loss is affected differently than someone with the same hearing thresholds who also has significant visual or mobility impairments.

Nevertheless, some basic scheme for classifying the severity of hearing loss is necessary. Although there is no universally accepted method for defining the degree of hearing loss, the following system is generally representative of various schemes currently in use:

- **0–25 dB**: Normal hearing.
- **26–40 dB**: Mild hearing loss.
- **41–55 dB**: Moderate hearing loss.
- **56–70 dB**: Moderately severe hearing loss.
- **71–90 dB**: Severe hearing loss.
- **91+ dB**: Profound hearing loss.

LATERALITY OF HEARING LOSS

Hearing losses may be classified as either unilateral (affecting only one ear) or bilateral (affecting both ears). Bilateral hearing losses may be symmetric (approximately the same in each ear) or asymmetric (worse in one ear than the other). Hearing losses from environmental causes (such as noise, ototoxic chemicals, and aging) are generally bilateral and symmetric. In contrast, hearing losses from medical causes (such as ear infections, mumps, and acoustic tumors) are often unilateral or asymmetric. A substantial difference in hearing sensitivity between ears can, therefore, indicate a medically significant condition.[1]

Section 2.2 | Hearing Loss in Infants and Children

HEARING LOSS

Hearing loss can affect a child's ability to develop speech, language, and social skills. The earlier that children with hearing loss start receiving services, the more likely they are to reach their full potential. If you think that a child might have hearing loss, ask the child's doctor for a hearing screening as soon as possible. Do not wait!

WHAT IT IS

A hearing loss can occur when any part of the ear is not functioning in the usual way. This includes the outer ear, middle ear, inner ear, hearing (acoustic) nerve, and auditory system.

SIGNS AND SYMPTOMS

The signs and symptoms of hearing loss vary for each child. If you suspect that your child might have hearing loss, ask the child's doctor for a hearing screening as soon as possible. Don't wait!

---

[1] "Audiometry Procedures," Centers for Disease Control and Prevention (CDC), December 2019. Available online. URL: wwwn.cdc.gov/nchs/data/nhanes/2019-2020/manuals/2019-Audiometry-Procedures-Manual-508.pdf. Accessed October 10, 2024.

Even if a child has passed a hearing screening before, it is important to look for the following signs:

Signs in Babies
- Does not startle at loud noises.
- Does not turn to the source of a sound after six months of age.
- Does not say single words, such as "dada" or "mama," by one year of age.
- Turns their head when they see you but does not respond if you only call their name. This may sometimes be mistaken for not paying attention or ignoring, but it could indicate partial or complete hearing loss.
- Seems to hear some sounds but not others.

Signs in Children
- Speech is delayed.
- Speech is not clear.
- Does not follow directions. This may also be mistaken for not paying attention or ignoring, but could indicate partial or complete hearing loss.
- Often says, "Huh?"
- Turns the TV or radio volume up too high.

CAUSES
Hearing loss can happen at any time during life—from before birth to adulthood.

The following factors can increase the likelihood of a child having hearing loss:
- **Genetic causes.** About one in two cases of hearing loss in babies is due to genetic factors. Some babies with a genetic cause for their hearing loss might have family members who also experience hearing loss. About one in three babies with genetic hearing loss have a "syndrome," meaning they have other conditions in addition to the hearing loss, such as Down syndrome or Usher syndrome.

- **Maternal infections and complications.** Approximately, one in four cases of hearing loss in babies is due to maternal infections during pregnancy, complications after birth, or head trauma. For example, the child:
  - was exposed to infection, such as during pregnancy
  - spent five days or more in a hospital neonatal intensive care unit (NICU) or had complications while in the NICU
  - needed a special procedure, such as a blood transfusion, to treat severe jaundice
  - has head, face, or ears shaped or formed differently than usual
  - has a condition such as a neurological disorder associated with hearing loss
  - had an infection around the brain and spinal cord called "meningitis"
  - received a significant head injury that required a hospital stay

PREVENTION
Parents can take the following steps to help prevent hearing loss in their children:
- Have a healthy pregnancy.
- Ensure that your child receives all childhood vaccines on schedule.
- Keep your child away from high noise levels, such as from very loud toys.

SCREENING AND DIAGNOSIS
Hearing screening can identify whether a child might have hearing loss. It is easy and painless, and babies are often asleep during the procedure, which usually takes only a few minutes.

Babies
All babies should have a hearing screening no later than one month of age. Most babies are screened while still in the hospital after birth. If a baby does not pass a hearing screening, it is crucial to get a full hearing test as soon as possible, ideally no later than three months of age.

Children

Children should have their hearing tested before they enter school or any time there is a concern about their hearing. Children who do not pass the hearing screening need to have a full hearing test as soon as possible.

TREATMENT

No single treatment or intervention is suitable for every person or family. Good treatment plans will include close monitoring, follow-ups, and any necessary adjustments along the way. There are many types of communication options for children with hearing loss and their families, including:
- learning alternative communication methods, such as sign language
- utilizing technology to assist with communication, such as hearing aids and cochlear implants
- using medicine and surgery to correct certain types of hearing loss
- accessing family support services

GET HELP

- If you think that your child might have hearing loss, ask the child's doctor for a hearing screening as soon as possible. Do not wait!
- If your child does not pass a hearing screening, request a full hearing test from the child's doctor as soon as possible.
- If your child has hearing loss, talk to the child's doctor about treatment and intervention services.

Early identification and intervention for hearing loss are crucial for a child's development. By recognizing the signs and seeking timely screening and treatment, families can support their child's speech, language, and social skills.[1]

---

[1] "About Hearing Loss in Children," Centers for Disease Control and Prevention (CDC), May 15, 2024. Available online. URL: www.cdc.gov/hearing-loss-children/about. Accessed October 3, 2024.

Section 2.3 | Hearing Loss in Older Adults

HEARING LOSS

Hearing loss is a common problem caused by loud noise, aging, disease, and genetic variations. About one-third of older adults experience hearing loss, and the chance of developing hearing loss increases with age. People with hearing loss may find it challenging to have conversations with friends and family. They may also have difficulty understanding a doctor's advice, responding to warnings, and hearing doorbells and alarms.

Some individuals may be reluctant to admit they have trouble hearing. Ignoring or leaving hearing problems untreated can lead to worsening conditions. If you have a hearing problem, consult your doctor. Hearing aids, special training, certain medications, and surgery are some of the treatments that can help.

SIGNS OF HEARING LOSS

Some people have a hearing problem and may not realize it. You should see your doctor if you meet any of the following criteria:
- Have trouble understanding what people are saying over the telephone.
- Find it hard to follow conversations when two or more people are talking.
- Often ask people to repeat what they are saying.
- Need to turn up the TV volume to a level that others complain about.
- Have difficulty understanding speech because of background noise.
- Think that others seem to mumble.
- Cannot understand what is being said when children or individuals with higher-pitched voices speak to you.

TYPES OF HEARING LOSS

Hearing loss comes in many forms and can range from mild loss, where a person misses certain high-pitched sounds, to total loss of hearing.

Sudden Hearing Loss
Sudden deafness, also known as "sudden sensorineural hearing loss," is an unexplained rapid loss of hearing. It can happen all at once or over a period of a few days and should be considered a medical emergency. If you or someone you know experiences sudden hearing loss, visit a doctor immediately.

Age-Related Hearing Loss
Age-related hearing loss, also called "presbycusis," develops gradually as a person ages. It often runs in families and may occur due to changes in the inner ear and auditory nerve. Presbycusis may make it hard for a person to tolerate loud sounds or understand what others are saying.

Age-related hearing loss usually affects both ears equally. Because the loss is gradual, people with presbycusis may not realize they have lost some of their hearing ability.

Tinnitus
Tinnitus is common in older people and is typically described as ringing in the ears, although it can also sound like roaring, clicking, hissing, or buzzing. It may come and go, can be heard in one or both ears, and may be loud or soft. Tinnitus is sometimes the first sign of hearing loss in older adults and can accompany any type of hearing loss.

Tinnitus is a symptom, not a disease. Something as simple as a piece of earwax blocking the ear canal can cause it. Tinnitus can also be a sign of other health conditions, such as high blood pressure (HBP) or allergies, and may occur as a side effect of certain medications.

CAUSES OF HEARING LOSS
- **Loud noise is one of the most common causes of hearing loss.** Noise from lawnmowers, snow blowers, or loud music can damage the inner ear and lead to permanent hearing loss. Loud noise also contributes to tinnitus. Most noise-related hearing loss can be prevented by turning down the sound on devices, moving away from loud noise, or using earplugs or other ear protection.

- **Earwax or fluid buildup can also cause hearing loss by blocking sounds carried from the eardrum to the inner ear.** If wax blockage is a problem, your doctor may suggest mild treatments to soften the earwax.
- **A ruptured eardrum can also cause hearing loss.** The eardrum can be damaged by infection, pressure, or inserting objects into the ear, including cotton-tipped swabs. Consult your doctor if you experience ear pain or fluid draining from the ear.
- **Health conditions common in older adults, such as diabetes or HBP, can contribute to hearing loss.** Ear infections caused by viruses and bacteria (also known as "otitis media" (OM)), heart conditions, strokes, brain injuries, or tumors may also affect hearing.
- **Hearing loss can also result from taking certain medications that can damage the inner ear, sometimes permanently.** These medications may be used to treat serious infections, cancer, or heart disease and include some antibiotics and even aspirin at certain dosages. If you notice a hearing problem while taking medication, consult your doctor.
- **Genetic variations can also cause hearing loss.** Not all inherited forms of hearing loss are evident at birth; some may develop later in life. For example, otosclerosis, thought to be a hereditary disease, involves abnormal bone growth that prevents structures within the ear from functioning properly.

HEALTH EFFECTS OF HEARING LOSS

Hearing loss can affect cognitive health. Studies have shown that older adults with hearing loss have a greater risk of developing dementia than older adults with normal hearing. Cognitive abilities (including memory and concentration) decline faster in older adults with hearing loss compared to their peers with normal hearing. A recent analysis of several studies found that individuals who used hearing restorative devices (such as hearing aids and cochlear implants) had a lower risk of long-term cognitive decline compared to those with uncorrected hearing loss.

Older people who cannot hear well may become depressed or withdrawn from others due to frustration or embarrassment about not understanding conversations. Sometimes, older individuals are mistakenly perceived as confused, unresponsive, or uncooperative because of their hearing difficulties. These circumstances can lead to social isolation and loneliness.

Even small amounts of hearing loss are linked to an increased risk of falls. It can also affect public and personal safety, such as the ability to drive safely when warning sounds are harder to hear.

HOW TO COPE WITH HEARING LOSS

If you notice signs of hearing loss, talk with your doctor. If you have trouble hearing, you should take the following steps:

- **Inform your family and friends**. Let your family and friends know about your hearing problem.
- **Ask people to face you and speak louder and more clearly**. Request them to repeat themselves or rephrase what they are saying.
- **Pay attention to what is being said and to facial expressions or gestures**.
- **Clarify what you do not understand**. Inform the speaker if you do not understand what was said.
- **Find a suitable location for conversation**. Position yourself between the speaker and sources of noise or look for quieter places to talk.

The most important action you can take if you think you have a hearing problem is to seek professional advice. Your family doctor may be able to diagnose and treat your hearing issue or refer you to other experts, such as an otolaryngologist (ear, nose, and throat doctor) or an audiologist (a health professional who can identify and measure hearing loss).

DEVICES TO HELP WITH HEARING LOSS

Many types of assistive devices are available to help people with hearing loss. These devices can amplify sounds, provide alerts, and assist in communication. For example, alert systems work with doorbells, smoke detectors, and alarm clocks to send visual signals or vibrations. Devices that utilize keyboards, touch screens, or text-to-speech technology can help you give and receive information more effectively.

Hearing Aids

Hearing aids are electronic, battery-operated assistive devices that make certain sounds louder. There are two main ways to acquire a hearing aid: by prescription or over the counter (OTC).

An audiologist or hearing aid specialist can prescribe hearing aids for individuals with significant or complicated hearing loss. Prescription hearing aids require a medical exam, after which the health-care professional will fit and adjust the device.

Hearing aids are now available without a prescription. OTC hearing aids, sold in stores and online, may help individuals with mild to moderate hearing loss. Before purchasing a hearing aid, find out if your health insurance will cover part of the cost.

Cochlear Implant

A cochlear implant is a different type of assistive device designed to help individuals who are profoundly deaf or hard of hearing. Whereas hearing aids amplify sound for damaged ears, cochlear implants create electric signals that the brain recognizes as sound. The implant requires surgical placement and hearing therapy.

If you are experiencing hearing loss, talk with your doctor about assistive devices that may be available to help.

HOW TO COMMUNICATE WITH SOMEONE WHO HAS HEARING LOSS

Here are some tips for communicating effectively with someone who has a hearing problem:
- In a group, make a point to include individuals with hearing loss in the conversation.
- Find a quiet place to talk to help reduce background noise, especially in restaurants and at social gatherings.
- Stand in good lighting and use facial expressions or gestures to provide visual cues.

- Face the person and speak clearly while maintaining eye contact.
- Speak a little louder than normal, but do not shout.
- Try to speak naturally and at a reasonable pace.
- Avoid hiding your mouth, eating, or chewing gum while speaking.
- Repeat yourself if necessary, using different words.
- Ensure that only one person talks at a time.
- Ask how you can help.[1]

---

[1] National Institute on Aging (NIA), "Hearing Loss: A Common Problem for Older Adults," National Institutes of Health (NIH), January 19, 2023. Available online. URL: www.nia.nih.gov/health/hearing-and-hearing-loss/hearing-loss-common-problem-older-adults. Accessed October 3, 2024.

Chapter 3 | **Auditory Impairment and Quality of Life**

Chapter Contents
Section 3.1—Effects of Hearing Loss on Daily Life and Well-Being...........24
Section 3.2—Barriers to Accessibility and Participation....................26
Section 3.3—Addressing Communication Needs in Auditory Impairment 30

Section 3.1 | Effects of Hearing Loss on Daily Life and Well-Being

Hearing loss is common in the United States. More people experience hearing loss than diabetes, cancer, or vision problems. Occupational hearing loss, caused by exposure to loud noise or chemicals that damage hearing at work, is the most prevalent work-related illness and is often permanent.

CONSEQUENCES OF HEARING LOSS

Hearing loss can profoundly affect the quality of life. The effects begin small and progress as hearing loss worsens. For most individuals, it starts with others sounding like they are mumbling because some sounds cannot be heard well. The individual often has to ask others to repeat themselves, leading to frustration for both parties. Consequently, both may limit the length and depth of conversations. As hearing loss progresses, it becomes increasingly difficult to hear others in the presence of background noise. Social gatherings and even dining at a restaurant become isolating experiences due to the inability to understand conversations, hindering participation. Over time, these communication barriers can lead to strained marriages, diminished or lost friendships, and limited interactions with coworkers and supervisors.

EFFECTS ON ENJOYMENT AND DAILY LIFE

Other effects include a loss of enjoyment in life. Sounds such as music, forest sounds, and a grandchild's voice become muted and lack quality. Even a person with mild hearing loss has trouble hearing softer sounds, struggles to differentiate between the softest and loudest sounds, and experiences increased listening fatigue. To compensate for this loss of sensitivity, people with hearing loss often need to "turn it up" whenever possible. Having the TV and radio at high volume can annoy others, leading a spouse or roommate to choose to watch TV in another room, thus transforming a group activity into a solo one.

SAFETY CONCERNS

Safety can also be compromised. Sounds like a tea kettle boiling, the warning beep of a forklift backing up, or the engine of an oncoming car may go unnoticed. There can be a general loss of situational awareness, and it is well known that workers with hearing loss are more likely to be injured on the job.

MENTAL HEALTH IMPLICATIONS

Not surprisingly, all these challenges can affect a person's mental health. Hearing loss is strongly associated with depression. Individuals with depression are also less likely to engage in activities with others, leading to compounded effects of hearing loss and depression that intensify isolation. Additionally, hearing loss is associated with cognitive decline, which includes memory and thinking skills loss. As individuals lose their ability to hear, they do not utilize the hearing-related parts of their brains as much, leading to deterioration in those areas. This illustrates the concept of "use it or lose it."

Often, those with hearing loss also experience "ringing in the ears" (tinnitus). Tinnitus can manifest as an annoying buzzing, rushing, or ringing noise in the ears or head. For some individuals, tinnitus can be more than just annoying; it can disrupt sleep and concentration, increasing fatigue and affecting alertness. The symptoms can be intermittent or continuous. Like hearing loss, tinnitus can influence mental health and is associated with depression and anxiety.

QUANTIFYING THE CONSEQUENCES OF HEARING LOSS

One way to measure the consequences of hearing loss on critical intangibles, such as communication and mental health, is to calculate disability-adjusted life years (DALYs). DALYs represent the number of healthy years lost due to a disease or health condition. In the case of hearing loss, it does not imply that a person dies younger; rather, it indicates fewer years of good health. The DALYs calculation takes into account life limitations caused by hearing loss as a lost portion of a healthy year of life, ultimately yielding the number of healthy years lost by a group of people over a specific time period.[1]

---

[1] "Measuring the Impact of Hearing Loss on Quality of Life," Centers for Disease Control and Prevention (CDC), April 27, 2016. Available online. URL: https://blogs.cdc.gov/niosh-science-blog/2016/04/27/hearing-loss-years-lost. Accessed October 5, 2024.

Section 3.2 | Barriers to Accessibility and Participation

Nearly everyone faces hardships and difficulties at some point in their lives. However, for people with disabilities, barriers can be more frequent and have a greater effect. The World Health Organization's (WHO) definition of barriers is as follows:

> Factors in a person's environment that, through their absence or presence, limit functioning and create disability. These include aspects such as:
> - A physical environment that is not accessible.
> - Lack of relevant assistive technology (assistive, adaptive, and rehabilitative devices).
> - Negative attitudes of people toward disability.
> - Services, systems, and policies that are either nonexistent or that hinder the involvement of all people with a health condition in all areas of life.

Often, multiple barriers can make it extremely difficult, or even impossible, for people with disabilities to function. Here are the seven most common barriers, which often occur concurrently:
1. attitudinal
2. communication
3. physical
4. policy
5. programmatic
6. social
7. transportation

ATTITUDINAL BARRIERS

Attitudinal barriers are the most basic and contribute to other barriers. For example, some people may not realize that difficulties in accessing places can limit a person with a disability from participating in everyday activities. Examples of attitudinal barriers include:
- **Stereotyping**. Some people stereotype those with disabilities, assuming their quality of life is poor or that they are unhealthy because of their impairments.

- **Stigma, prejudice, and discrimination.** Within society, these attitudes may stem from misconceptions related to disability. People may view disability as a personal tragedy, as something that needs to be cured or prevented, as a punishment for wrongdoing, or as an indication of a lack of ability to behave as expected in society.

Today, society's understanding of disability is improving, recognizing that "disability" occurs when a person's functional needs are not addressed in their physical and social environment. By reframing disability as a social responsibility, it becomes easier to identify and address the challenges that all people—especially those with disabilities—experience.

COMMUNICATION BARRIERS
Communication barriers are encountered by people who have disabilities affecting hearing, speaking, reading, writing, or understanding, and who use different ways to communicate than those who do not have these disabilities. Examples of communication barriers include:
- Written health promotion messages with barriers that prevent people with vision impairments from receiving the message, such as:
  - use of small print without large-print versions
  - lack of Braille or versions for people who use screen readers
- Auditory health messages may be inaccessible to people with hearing impairments, including:
  - videos that do not include captioning
  - oral communications without accompanying manual interpretation (e.g., American Sign Language (ASL))
- The use of technical language, long sentences, and polysyllabic words can create significant barriers to understanding for people with cognitive impairments.

PHYSICAL BARRIERS
Physical barriers are structural obstacles in natural or human-made environments that impede mobility (the ability to move around in the environment) or access. Examples of physical barriers include:
- steps and curbs that prevent individuals with mobility impairments from entering a building or using a sidewalk
- mammography equipment that requires women with mobility impairments to stand
- the absence of a weight scale that accommodates wheelchairs or individuals who have difficulty stepping up

POLICY BARRIERS
Policy barriers often relate to a lack of awareness or enforcement of existing laws and regulations that require programs and activities to be accessible to people with disabilities. Examples of policy barriers include:
- denying qualified individuals with disabilities the opportunity to participate in or benefit from federally funded programs, services, or other benefits
- denying individuals with disabilities access to programs, services, benefits, or opportunities to participate due to physical barriers
- denying reasonable accommodations to qualified individuals with disabilities so they can perform the essential functions of the job for which they have applied or have been hired

PROGRAMMATIC BARRIERS
Programmatic barriers limit the effective delivery of public health or health-care programs for people with different types of impairments. Examples of programmatic barriers include:
- inconvenient scheduling
- lack of accessible equipment (e.g., mammography screening equipment)
- insufficient time allocated for medical examinations and procedures
- little or no communication with patients or participants
- provider attitudes, knowledge, and understanding of people with disabilities

SOCIAL BARRIERS

Social barriers relate to the conditions in which people are born, grow, live, learn, work, and age—known as "social determinants of health" (SDOH)—that can contribute to decreased functioning among people with disabilities. Examples of social barriers include the following:

- **Employment disparities.** People with disabilities are far less likely to be employed. In 2017, 35.5 percent of people with disabilities aged 18–64 were employed, compared to 76.5 percent of individuals without disabilities.
- **Educational attainment.** Adults aged 18 years and older with disabilities are less likely to have completed high school compared to their peers without disabilities (22.3% vs. 10.1%).
- **Income inequality.** People with disabilities are more likely to have an income of less than $15,000 compared to those without disabilities (22.3% vs. 7.3%).
- **Increased risk of violence.** Children with disabilities are almost four times more likely to experience violence than children without disabilities.

TRANSPORTATION BARRIERS

Transportation barriers arise from a lack of adequate transportation, which interferes with an individual's ability to be independent and function in society. Examples of transportation barriers include:

- lack of access to accessible or convenient transportation
- unavailable or inconveniently located public transportation

By recognizing these challenges, we can work toward creating solutions that enhance accessibility and promote equal opportunities for everyone.[1]

---

[1] National Center on Birth Defects and Developmental Disabilities (NCBDDD), "Disability Barriers to Inclusion," Centers for Disease Control and Prevention (CDC), May 2, 2024. Available online. URL: www.cdc.gov/ncbddd/disabilityandhealth/disability-barriers.html. Accessed October 7, 2024.

Section 3.3 | Addressing Communication Needs in Auditory Impairment

PREVALENCE OF HEARING LOSS

Hearing loss is prevalent in the United States, with at least 20 percent of U.S. adults experiencing significant difficulty with hearing, balance, taste, smell, voice, speech, or language at some point in their lives. These challenges can compromise physical and emotional health and affect social, educational, vocational, and recreational aspects of life.

Hearing loss and other communication disorders can affect individuals at any age. For example, hearing loss can be present at birth or develop over time, while voice, speech, or language disorders can affect various groups, including children with autism spectrum disorder, people who stutter, and adults who rely heavily on their voices for work, such as teachers and performers.

Hearing loss and voice, speech, and language disorders can be particularly challenging for young children and older adults. Hearing problems in children can delay the development of voice, speech, and language skills. Additionally, children with developmental speech and language problems are at risk for learning disabilities and psychosocial issues that may emerge during adolescence or adulthood.

Some communication disorders are associated with other conditions. For example, aphasia, which affects the ability to speak, write, and understand language, often results from brain damage, most commonly due to a stroke. Although people of any age can acquire aphasia, the disorder most frequently affects adults who are middle-aged or older.

One of the most common communication disorders in older adults is hearing loss, affecting approximately one in three adults aged 65–74 and nearly half of those older than 75. Hearing loss can lead to feelings of isolation and a loss of connection with family, friends, and the community. Although hearing aids and other assistive devices can improve quality of life, only about one in four adults (aged 20 and over) who could benefit from hearing aids has ever used them.[1]

LAWS PERTAINING TO EFFECTIVE COMMUNICATION FOR INDIVIDUALS WHO ARE DEAF OR HARD OF HEARING
Section 504
Section 504 of the Rehabilitation Act of 1973 (Section 504) prohibits public and private entities that receive financial assistance from any federal department or agency (covered entities) from excluding qualified individuals with disabilities or denying them an equal opportunity to receive program benefits and services.

ADA
The Americans with Disabilities Act of 1990 (ADA) protects individuals with disabilities in employment, state and local government services, public accommodations (most private offices and businesses), transportation, and telecommunications.

WHO ARE PROTECTED UNDER THESE LAWS?
These laws protect qualified individuals with disabilities who meet the following criteria:
- Have a physical or mental impairment that substantially limits one or more major life activities (such as hearing, speaking, sleeping, thinking, learning, working, or the operation of a major bodily function).
- Have a record of such an impairment.
- Are regarded as having such an impairment.

To receive services, education, or training, qualified individuals with disabilities must—with or without reasonable modifications—meet the essential eligibility requirements for the specific service, program, or activity.

---

[1] "Communication Is Key at All Ages: Learn More during Better Hearing and Speech Month," National Institute on Deafness and Other Communication Disorders (NIDCD), February 23, 2023. Available online. URL: www.nidcd.nih.gov/news/2019/may-is-better-hearing-and-speech-month. Accessed October 5, 2024.

Examples
- A 40-year-old person who is deaf would not qualify for a program limited to individuals over 65.
- A seven-year-old child who is hard of hearing would likely qualify for a vaccination program provided to all school-age children.

WHAT ARE AUXILIARY AIDS AND SERVICES?
Auxiliary aids and services may include:
- qualified interpreters (who can interpret effectively, accurately, and impartially, both receptively and expressively, using any necessary specialized vocabulary)
- note takers
- transcription services
- written materials
- telephone handset amplifiers
- assistive listening devices and systems
- telephones compatible with hearing aids
- closed caption decoders and open and closed captioning
- text telephones
- videotext displays or other effective methods of making aurally delivered materials (information delivered through sound, including speech, intercoms, telephones, recorded messages, loudspeakers, alarms, etc.) available to individuals who are deaf or hard of hearing

WHAT SHOULD YOU DO IF YOU NEED AUXILIARY AID OR SERVICE?
As soon as possible:
1. Inform the entity that you are deaf or hard of hearing.
2. Request the auxiliary aid or service you believe you need (interpreter, notepaper, etc.).

WHO DECIDES ON THE AID OR SERVICE?
The covered entity is responsible for ensuring effective communication.

Auditory Impairment and Quality of Life | 33

Generally, the entity should consult with you and give primary consideration to fulfilling your request. They may use a substitute if the alternative also provides effective communication. If an auxiliary aid or service is needed, the entity must provide it free of charge after considering the following:
- The number of people participating in the communication and their individual characteristics.
- The particular situation or context, including the nature, length, complexity, and importance of the communication.
- Whether providing the aid or service would fundamentally alter the program or service or result in an undue burden. This decision must be made on a case-by-case basis.

Example Scenario

A person who is deaf visited the doctor's office for a blood test. The doctor knew that the visit would be short and that there would be minimal communication. After consulting with the individual, the doctor determined that an interpreter was not needed; instead, writing notes and gestures would be effective for this patient. However, for the next appointment to discuss the blood test results and treatment decisions, the doctor provided an interpreter. In making these decisions, the doctor consulted with the individual, considered their needs, and evaluated the circumstances, importance, and complexity of the communication, as well as whether providing an interpreter would constitute an undue burden under the law.

WHAT IF YOU THINK THE COMMUNICATION IS NOT EFFECTIVE?

You can inform the service provider if you believe that the communication is not or will not be effective. You should explain why you think it is inadequate.

Example Scenario

A parent with deafness who has a child in a Head Start program requested a meeting with the Director to discuss issues with the child's teacher. The Director asked a teacher who was a close friend of the child's teacher to serve as an interpreter. The parent expressed concerns that an outside interpreter should be obtained, as the chosen interpreter might not be able to remain impartial.[2]

---

[2] "Effective Communication for Persons Who Are Deaf or Hard of Hearing," U.S. Department of Health and Human Services (HHS), June 16, 2017. Available online. URL: www.hhs.gov/civil-rights/for-individuals/disability/effective-communication/index.html. Accessed October 5, 2024.

Chapter 4 | Communicating with People with Hearing Loss

Chapter Contents
Section 4.1—American Sign Language 36
Section 4.2—Telecommunications Relay Service 38

Section 4.1 | American Sign Language

WHAT IS AMERICAN SIGN LANGUAGE?
American Sign Language (ASL) is a complete, natural language with linguistic properties similar to spoken languages, though its grammar differs from English. ASL is expressed through movements of the hands and face. It serves as the primary language for many North Americans who are deaf or hard of hearing and is also used by some hearing people.

IS SIGN LANGUAGE THE SAME IN OTHER COUNTRIES?
There is no universal sign language. Different sign languages are used in various countries or regions. For example, British Sign Language (BSL) is distinct from ASL, meaning that Americans familiar with ASL may not understand BSL. Some countries incorporate features of ASL into their sign languages.

WHERE DID AMERICAN SIGN LANGUAGE ORIGINATE?
No single person or committee invented ASL. The exact origins of ASL are unclear, but some suggest it arose more than 200 years ago from the intermixing of local sign languages and French Sign Language (Langue des Signes Française, or LSF). Today's ASL includes elements of LSF and the original local sign languages, which have evolved into a rich, complex, and mature language. Modern ASL and LSF are now distinct languages; while they still share some signs, they are no longer mutually intelligible.

HOW DOES AMERICAN SIGN LANGUAGE COMPARE WITH SPOKEN LANGUAGE?
American Sign Language is entirely separate and distinct from English. It has all the fundamental features of language, including its own rules for pronunciation, word formation, and word order. While every language has methods of signaling different functions, such as asking a question instead of making a statement, these methods differ across languages. For example, English speakers might ask a question by raising the pitch of their voices and adjusting

word order, whereas ASL users ask a question by raising their eyebrows, widening their eyes, and tilting their bodies forward.

As with other languages, the ways of expressing ideas in ASL vary among its users. In addition to individual differences in expression, ASL features regional accents and dialects. Just as certain English words are pronounced differently in various parts of the country, ASL exhibits regional variations in signing rhythm, pronunciation, slang, and the signs used. Other sociological factors, including age and gender, also influence ASL usage and contribute to its variety, similar to spoken languages.

Finger spelling is an integral part of ASL and is used to spell out English words. In the finger-spelled alphabet, each letter corresponds to a distinct handshape. Finger spelling is often employed for proper names or to indicate the English word for something.

HOW DO MOST CHILDREN LEARN AMERICAN SIGN LANGUAGE?

Parents are typically the primary source of a child's early language acquisition, but for children who are deaf, additional people may serve as language models. A child with deafness born to parents who also have deafness and already use ASL will naturally acquire ASL, much like a hearing child learns spoken language from hearing parents. However, for a child with deafness and hearing parents who have no prior experience with ASL, language acquisition may differ. In fact, 9 out of 10 children born deaf have hearing parents. Some hearing parents choose to introduce sign language to their children with deafness, learning it alongside them. Children with deafness and hearing parents often learn sign language through deaf peers and become fluent over time.

WHY EMPHASIZE EARLY LANGUAGE LEARNING?

It is essential for parents to expose a child who is deaf or hard of hearing to language (spoken or signed) as early as possible. The sooner a child is exposed to and begins to acquire language, the better their language, cognitive, and social development will be. Research indicates that the first few years of life are critical for language skill development, with even the early months being vital for establishing effective communication with caregivers. Due to screening programs in place at almost all hospitals in the United States and its territories, newborns are tested for hearing before leaving the hospital. If a baby has hearing loss, this screening allows parents to learn about communication options and start their child's language learning process during this crucial early stage of development (www.nidcd.nih.gov/health/your-babys-hearing-screening-and-next-steps#8).[1]

Section 4.2 | Telecommunications Relay Service

ACCESS TO TELECOMMUNICATIONS RELAY SERVICES

Telecommunications Relay Service (TRS) allows people with hearing or speech disabilities to place and receive telephone calls. TRS is available in all 50 states, the District of Columbia, Puerto Rico, and U.S. territories for local and/or long-distance calls.

TRS providers are compensated for the costs of providing TRS from either a state or a federal fund. Internet Protocol (IP) Relay is not mandated by the Federal Communications Commission (FCC).

TRS providers must ensure user confidentiality, and Communications Assistants (CAs), with a limited exception for Speech-to-Speech (STS), may not keep records of the contents of any conversation. Users of Voice over Internet Protocol (VoIP) services can also access relay services by dialing 711.

WHAT FORMS OF TELECOMMUNICATIONS RELAY SERVICES ARE AVAILABLE?

There are several forms of TRS, depending on the particular needs of the user and the equipment available:
- **Text-to-Voice TTY-based TRS.** This "traditional" TRS service uses a TTY (teletypewriter) to call the CA at the relay center. TTYs have a keyboard that allows users to

---

[1] "American Sign Language," National Institute on Deafness and Other Communication Disorders (NIDCD), October 29, 2021. Available online. URL: www.nidcd.nih.gov/health/american-sign-language. Accessed October 5, 2024.

Communicating with People with Hearing Loss | 39

type their telephone conversations. The text is displayed on a screen or printed on paper. A TTY user calls a TRS relay center and types the number of the person they wish to call. The CA at the relay center then makes a voice telephone call to the other party and relays the conversation by speaking what the text user types and typing what the voice telephone user speaks.
- **Voice Carry Over (VCO)**. This service allows a person with a hearing disability who wants to use their own voice to speak directly to the called party while receiving responses in text from the CA. No typing is required by the calling party. This service is particularly useful for senior citizens who have lost their hearing but can still speak.
- **Hearing Carry Over (HCO)**. This service allows a person with a speech disability, but who can use their own hearing, to listen to the called party while typing their part of the conversation on a TTY. The CA reads these words to the called party, and the caller hears responses directly from the called party.
- **Speech-to-Speech Relay Service (STS)**. This service is used by a person with a speech disability. A CA, specially trained in understanding a variety of speech disorders, repeats what the caller says in a manner that makes the caller's words clear and understandable to the called party. No special telephone is needed. For more information, visit the STS Relay Service consumer guide (www.fcc.gov/consumers/guides/speech-speech-relay-service).
- **Shared Non-English Language Relay Services**. Due to the large number of Spanish speakers in the United States, the FCC requires interstate TRS providers to offer Spanish-to-Spanish traditional TRS. Although Spanish language relay is not mandated for intrastate (within a state) TRS, many states with large populations of Spanish speakers offer this service on a voluntary basis. The FCC also allows TRS providers who voluntarily offer other shared non-English language interstate TRS, such as French-to-French, to be compensated from the federal TRS fund.

- **Captioned Telephone Service.** This service is used by people with a hearing disability who have some residual hearing. It employs a special telephone with a text screen to display captions of what the other party is saying. A captioned telephone allows the user to speak to the called party while simultaneously listening and reading captions of the conversation. There is also a "two-line" version of captioned telephone service that offers additional features, such as call-waiting, *69, call forwarding, and direct dialing for 911 emergency services. Unlike traditional TRS, where the CA types what the called party says, the CA repeats or re-voices what the called party says. Speech recognition technology automatically transcribes the CA's voice into text, which is then transmitted directly to the user's captioned telephone display.
- **IP Captioned Telephone Service.** This service combines elements of captioned telephone service and IP Relay. IP captioned telephone service can be provided in various ways but uses the Internet rather than traditional telephone networks to provide the link and captions between the caller with a hearing disability and the CA. It allows the user to simultaneously listen to and read the text of what the other party is saying. IP captioned telephone service can be used with an existing voice telephone and a computer or other web-enabled device without requiring specialized equipment. For more information, visit the IP CTS consumer guide (www.fcc.gov/consumers/guides/internet-protocol-ip-captioned-telephone-service).
- **Internet Protocol Relay Service (IP Relay).** This text-based form of TRS uses the Internet, rather than traditional telephone lines, for the leg of the call between the person with a hearing or speech disability and the CA. Otherwise, the call is handled similarly to a TTY-based TRS call. The user may use a computer or other web-enabled device to communicate with the CA. IP Relay is not required by the FCC. For more information, visit the IP Relay Service consumer guide (www.fcc.gov/consumers/guides/ip-relay-service).

- **Video Relay Service (VRS).** This Internet-based form of TRS allows individuals whose primary language is American Sign Language (ASL) to communicate with the CA in ASL using video conferencing equipment. The CA speaks what is signed to the called party and signs the called party's response back to the caller. VRS is not required by the FCC, but it is offered by several TRS providers. VRS allows conversations to flow in near real-time and in a faster, more natural manner than text-based TRS. Beginning January 1, 2006, TRS providers that offer VRS must provide it 24 hours a day, seven days a week, and must answer incoming calls within a specific time frame to minimize wait times for VRS users. For more information, visit the VRS consumer guide (www.fcc.gov/consumers/guides/video-relay-services).

711 ACCESS TO TELECOMMUNICATIONS RELAY SERVICES

Just as you can call 411 for information, you can dial 711 to connect to certain forms of TRS anywhere in the United States. Dialing 711 makes it easier for travelers to use TRS because they do not have to remember TRS numbers for each state. However, 711 access is not available for Captioned Telephone Service (CTS), IP Captioned Telephone Service (IP CTS), Video Relay Service (VRS), or IP Relay. For more information, visit the 711 consumer guide (www.fcc.gov/consumers/guides/711-telecommunications-relay-service).[1]

---

[1] "Telecommunications Relay Service," Federal Communications Commission (FCC), August 16, 2022. Available online. URL: www.fcc.gov/consumers/guides/telecommunications-relay-service-trs. Accessed October 5, 2024.

Part 2 | Effect of Noise on Hearing Loss

Chapter 5 | **Noise-Induced Hearing Loss**

Many enjoyable sounds that we hear every day are at safe levels that would not damage our hearing. However, sounds can be harmful when they are too loud—even for a short time—or when they are long-lasting, even if they are not quite as loud. These sounds can damage part of the inner ear and cause permanent hearing loss, which can worsen over a lifetime.

PREVALENCE OF HEARING LOSS

Hearing loss from noise can happen to anyone at any age. Analyses from nationally representative health interviews and examination surveys found that about one in seven U.S. teens aged 12–19 (13–18%) and nearly one in four (24%) U.S. adults aged 20–69 have features of their hearing test in one or both ears that suggest noise-induced hearing loss.

MECHANISM OF HEARING

To understand how loud noises can damage our hearing, we must understand how we hear. Hearing depends on a series of complex steps that change sound waves in the air into electrical signals. The auditory nerve then carries these signals to the brain for us to understand.

Noise-induced hearing loss happens when tiny hair-like structures (stereocilia) that sit on top of hair cells in the inner ear are damaged by noises that are too loud and/or last for too long. When stereocilia are damaged, the hair cells cannot send information about the sound to the brain, leading to permanent hearing loss.

MEASURING SOUND

Sound is measured in units called "decibels" (dB). An increase of 10 dB seems about twice as loud to your ears, but it is actually

10 times more intense, or powerful! Because people cannot hear all frequencies, or pitches of sound, A-weighted decibels (dBA) can be used to describe sound based on what human ears can actually hear. A whisper is 30 dBA, and normal conversational speech is about 60–70 dBA.

The louder the sound, the shorter it takes for possible hearing loss to occur. For example, firecrackers are often 160 dBA and can cause hearing damage much more quickly than exposure to a power lawn mower at 80–100 dBA.

CAUSES AND EFFECTS OF HEARING LOSS

Hearing loss from noise can be caused by exposure to constant loud sounds over a long period of time, such as noise in a woodworking shop.

Many everyday activities can put children at risk for hearing loss caused by noise. These activities include:
- listening to music at high volume through earbuds or headphones
- playing in a band or orchestra
- attending loud concerts
- being around loud noises at home for a long period of time, such as lawnmowers or leaf blowers
- riding snowmobiles or motorcycles

Hearing loss caused by noise can be temporary. For some people, hearing returns to normal levels 16–48 hours after exposure to loud noises. Recent research suggests, however, that there may still be long-term, permanent damage even if it is not immediately noticeable or detectable.

SIGNS OF HEARING LOSS

Hearing loss due to loud noises can also build over time, so signs may not be readily noticeable. As hearing loss progresses, people might experience the following:
- Complain of ringing or buzzing in the ear—called "tinnitus." Tinnitus may go away over time, but it can sometimes continue for a long time or throughout a person's life.

- Say "What?" more often or ask others to repeat what they have said.
- Turn up the sound on the TV or other devices.

If you or someone you know regularly experiences any of these signs, you should get your hearing checked to determine if you have hearing loss.

GENETIC FACTORS OF HEARING LOSS

Although everyone is at risk for noise-induced hearing loss, some people may be at higher risk due to their genetics. Our genes, inherited from our parents, carry the information that forms the building blocks of who we are. Some people inherit genes that make them more likely to develop noise-induced hearing loss. Scientists are working to figure out which genes increase the risk.

PREVENTION STRATEGIES FOR HEARING LOSS

Hearing loss from noise can often be prevented. The best way to ensure that your children continue to enjoy the sounds they love throughout life is to teach them practical ways to protect their hearing. These include:
- lowering the volume
- moving away from the noise
- wearing hearing protectors, such as earplugs or earmuffs (If hearing protection is not available, cover your ears with your hands.)[1]

---

[1] "What Is Noise-Induced Hearing Loss?" National Institute on Deafness and Other Communication Disorders (NIDCD), June 3, 2019. Available online. URL: www.noisyplanet.nidcd.nih.gov/parents/what-is-noise-induced-hearing-loss. Accessed October 5, 2024.

Chapter 6 | **Workplace Noise**

Chapter Contents
Section 6.1—Effects of Workplace Noise on Hearing Health 50
Section 6.2—Occupational Noise Risks in Music and Aviation............... 51
Section 6.3—Hearing Loss in the Forestry and Logging Industry............ 53
Section 6.4—Effective Noise Reduction Techniques in the Workplace........ 56

Section 6.1 | Effects of Workplace Noise on Hearing Health

NOISE EXPOSURE AND ITS EFFECTS

Exposure to high levels of noise can cause permanent hearing loss. Neither surgery nor a hearing aid can help correct this type of hearing loss. Short-term exposure to loud noise can also cause a temporary change in hearing (your ears may feel stuffed up) or a ringing in your ears (tinnitus). These short-term problems may go away within a few minutes or hours after leaving the noisy environment. However, repeated exposure to loud noise can lead to permanent tinnitus and/or hearing loss.

Loud noise can create physical and psychological stress, reduce productivity, interfere with communication and concentration, and contribute to workplace accidents and injuries by making it difficult to hear warning signals. The effects of noise-induced hearing loss can be profound, limiting your ability to hear high-frequency sounds, understand speech, and seriously impairing your ability to communicate.

MEASURING EXPOSURE TO NOISE

Exposure to noise is measured in units of sound pressure levels called "decibels," using A-weighted sound levels (dBA). There are several ways to control and reduce worker exposure to noise in a workplace where exposure has been shown to be excessive.

ENGINEERING CONTROLS

Engineering controls involve modifying or replacing equipment or making related physical changes at the noise source or along the transmission path to reduce the noise level at the worker's ear. Examples of inexpensive, effective engineering controls include:
- choosing low-noise tools and machinery
- maintaining and lubricating machinery and equipment (e.g., oil bearings)
- placing a barrier between the noise source and the employee (e.g., sound walls or curtains)
- enclosing or isolating the noise source

ADMINISTRATIVE CONTROLS

Administrative controls are changes in the workplace or schedule that reduce or eliminate worker exposure to noise. Examples of noise control measures include the following:
- Operating noisy machines during shifts when fewer people are exposed.
- Limiting the amount of time a person spends at a noise source.
- Providing quiet areas where workers can gain relief from hazardous noise sources.
- Controlling noise exposure through distance, which is often an effective, yet simple and inexpensive administrative control. Specifically, for every doubling of the distance between the source of noise and the worker, the noise is decreased by 6 dBA.

REPORTING HEALTH AND SAFETY ISSUES

To discuss a health and safety issue at work, contact the Occupational Safety and Health Administration (OSHA) toll-free at 800-321-6742 or by email (www.osha.gov/form/ecorrespondence), or contact your nearest OSHA office (www.osha.gov/contactus/bystate). Your information will be kept confidential.[1]

Section 6.2 | Occupational Noise Risks in Music and Aviation

Hearing loss is one of the most common work-related illnesses in the United States. The National Institute for Occupational Safety and Health (NIOSH) estimates that 22 million U.S. workers encounter noise exposures loud enough to be hazardous, and the American Tinnitus Association estimates that 50 million Americans suffer from prolonged tinnitus.

---

[1] "Occupational Noise Exposure," Occupational Safety and Health Administration (OSHA), February 26, 2007. Available online. URL: www.osha.gov/noise/exposure-controls. Accessed October 5, 2024.

NOISE HAZARDS IN THE MUSIC INDUSTRY

Musicians and others involved in the music industry are at risk of developing permanent hearing loss, tinnitus (ringing in the ears), and other hearing disorders due to exposure to loud sounds.

As of 2012, the Bureau of Labor Statistics estimates that 167,400 people work as musicians and singers and 77,600 as music directors and composers. For professional musicians, hearing loss or tinnitus can significantly impair not only their communication and quality of life but also their career and ability to obtain or maintain a job.

Professional musicians work and practice in a variety of venues ranging from large music halls, theaters, and arenas to smaller clubs and school and university music rooms. Musicians are often overlooked in terms of occupational safety and health practices. Music-induced hearing loss occurs slowly and over a long period of time, and most musicians do not seek help until they start to experience secondary symptoms such as tinnitus (buzzing or ringing in the ears), distortion of sounds, diplacusis (hearing the same notes at different pitches), and hyperacusis (extreme sensitivity to everyday sounds).

In addition, negative health consequences are associated with producing high musical sound levels. Musicians are at increased risk for both musculoskeletal and vocal health problems when producing high sound levels on musical instruments such as the piano, trumpet, guitar, or drums. Increased biomechanical demands, whether at the hands, embouchure, or vocal cords, elevate the risks for occupational health problems such as tendonitis, carpal tunnel syndrome, rupture of facial muscles, and vocal cord malfunction.[1]

NOISE HAZARDS IN AVIATION

Occupational hearing loss is one of the most common work-related injuries in the United States. There are many sources of noise during flight operations. Talk to your employer and your health-care provider if you have concerns about your noise exposure at work.

---

[1] National Institute for Occupational Safety and Health (NIOSH), "Reducing the Risk of Hearing Disorders among Musicians," Centers for Disease Control and Prevention (CDC), June 2015. Available online. URL: www.cdc.gov/niosh/docs/wp-solutions/2015-184/pdfs/2015-184.pdf?id=10.26616/NIOSHPUB2015184. Accessed October 7, 2024.

On the ground, aircraft engines, takeoff preparations, and braking are sources of noise on aircraft.

When airborne, the aircraft engines and high-speed turbulence over the fuselage are the largest sources of noise on aircraft. Announcements and mechanical noises from food and beverage service are other sources of noise.

RECOMMENDED NOISE EXPOSURE LEVELS

The NIOSH recommends that all worker exposures to noise be controlled below a level equivalent to 85 dBA for eight hours to minimize occupational noise-induced hearing loss.

RECOMMENDATIONS FOR PROTECTION

Employers and employees can learn more about protecting employee hearing from the NIOSH Noise and Hearing Loss Prevention website (www.cdc.gov/niosh/noise/about/noise.html).

If you have concerns about your noise exposures, follow up with your health-care provider. You or your health-care provider may also contact CDC-INFO for more information (www.cdc.gov/cdc-info/index.html).[2]

Section 6.3 | Hearing Loss in the Forestry and Logging Industry

Hearing loss is common, especially among workers who are exposed to hazardous noise in their workplace. Noise is considered hazardous when it reaches 85 decibels (dBA) or more. In other words, when a person needs to raise his or her voice to speak with someone at arm's length or about 3 feet away, that person is likely being exposed to noise that can potentially damage his or her hearing over time. This exposure to hazardous noise and/or chemicals that

---

[2] National Institute for Occupational Safety and Health (NIOSH), "Aircrew and Aircrew and Noise," Centers for Disease Control and Prevention (CDC), September 11, 2024. Available online. URL: www.cdc.gov/niosh/aviation/prevention/aircrew-noise.html. Accessed October 7, 2024.

can damage hearing may lead to hearing loss linked to the workplace, also known as "occupational hearing loss."

INDUSTRY-SPECIFIC RISKS

The risk of developing hearing loss varies by industry. The National Institute for Occupational Safety and Health (NIOSH) recently examined one particular industry sector in its paper, *Prevalence of Hearing Loss Among Noise-Exposed Workers within the Agriculture, Forestry, Fishing, and Hunting Sector, 2003–2012*. This study looked at the number of workers in this industry sector who had a material hearing impairment, which is hearing loss that interferes with understanding speech.

Agriculture, Forestry, Fishing, and Hunting sector is among the top industry sectors for worker exposure to hazardous noise that can contribute to hearing loss (37% exposed versus 25% for all industries combined). Hearing loss within the forestry and logging industry is more pervasive. Noise-exposed workers in forestry and logging had a higher percentage of hearing loss (21%) than all noise-exposed industries combined (19%). To put this into perspective, a different study found that only 7 percent of non-noise-exposed workers reported hearing difficulty. Worker tasks in forestry and logging include:
- managing forest nurseries
- tending to timber tracts (plots of land selected for collecting timber)
- gathering forest products
- harvesting standing trees for timber

SOURCES OF HAZARDOUS NOISE

Activities associated with these tasks, such as unlatching cables used to hold and move logs (92 dBA) and the use of chainsaws (91–110 dBA), represent some of the highest noise exposures for this industry's workers. Overall average exposures in some occupations have been shown to range from 97 to 102 dBA. These noise exposures, among others, contribute to the elevated prevalence of hearing loss seen in this industry.

The highest prevalence of hearing loss (36%) was found in forest nurseries and the gathering of forest products within forestry and logging. This represents the highest prevalence within the Agriculture, Forestry, Fishing, and Hunting sector.

PREVENTION STRATEGIES IN FORESTRY AND LOGGING

Fortunately, there are effective methods for preventing worker hearing loss from noise. Reducing the noise, preferably at the source, is always the first and best step. To further reduce worker exposure to hazardous noise and minimize hearing loss within forestry and logging, this industry can implement the following measures:

- Enclose engines and heavy equipment workstations to contain the noise.
- Install silencers and mufflers on the equipment.
- Reduce exposure time for workers operating noisy equipment.
- Perform maintenance on hand tools and vehicle systems.
- Ensure that workers consistently wear properly fitted hearing protection every time they are in noisy areas or using noisy equipment.
- Make sure that employees receive regular monitoring for changes in their hearing so that additional measures to limit the progression of any detected hearing loss can be taken.

Forestry and logging activities can also expose workers to vibration, which may contribute to the risk of hearing loss through suspected changes to blood flow within the inner ear. Vibration exposure can be reduced through routine maintenance of equipment and the use of anti-vibration chainsaws and gloves.

HAND-ARM VIBRATION SYNDROME AND HEARING LOSS

It is important to limit noise and vibration at the source. When feasible, low-noise, low-vibration equipment should be provided and used. Sound and vibration level information can be found in manufacturers' product and technical brochures. If noisy or high-vibration equipment must be used, reducing the duration or number of tasks that require it can also decrease exposures. It is recommended that workers performing noisy or high-vibration tasks take breaks or are rotated periodically to other tasks that have lower exposures.

In addition, regularly maintaining tools and equipment according to manufacturers' recommendations can limit noise and vibration. Personal protective equipment, such as properly fitted earplugs and earmuffs, can reduce a worker's exposure to noise. For hand-arm vibration specifically, keeping hands warm and dry appears important in limiting vibration syndrome. For both hearing loss and vibration syndrome, it is essential that at-risk workers are educated about and monitored regularly for signs and symptoms.[1]

Section 6.4 | Effective Noise Reduction Techniques in the Workplace

Noise controls are often simple and easy to implement. They involve modifying equipment or making physical changes to the surrounding environment to reduce noise levels at the worker's ear. These controls are not always complex or costly; in fact, they can frequently be the most cost-effective solution. Implementing noise controls can lead to savings by reducing expenses related to hearing loss prevention programs, workers' compensation premiums, and hearing loss claims.

Before implementing noise controls, ensure that machinery is in good repair and that all maintenance procedures have been completed. In some cases, proper maintenance alone can effectively reduce noise to a safe level.

REDUCE SPEED OF MOVING PARTS

Parts or machinery that are in motion produce less sound energy at slower speeds. For example, slower fans with larger blades are quieter than smaller, faster fans moving the same volume of air.

---

[1] National Institute for Occupational Safety and Health (NIOSH), "Timber, Noise, and Hearing Loss: A Look into the Forestry and Logging Industry," Centers for Disease Control and Prevention (CDC), May 25, 2018. Available online. URL: https://blogs.cdc.gov/niosh-science-blog/2018/05/24/noise-forestry. Accessed October 8, 2024.

The same principle applies to noise generated by falling parts. The farther they fall, the more speed they gain, increasing the noise. To reduce noise from falling parts, decrease the falling distance.

ELIMINATE RESTRICTED FLOW IN PIPES OR DUCTS
Restricted flow in ducts and pipes can create additional turbulence, leading to increased noise levels. Removing obstructions such as flanges and valves can help reduce this noise.

ISOLATE MACHINE VIBRATION
Vibration isolation of machines can reduce excessive noise. When a vibrating machine is directly on the floor, it can cause noise in adjacent areas. Placing the machine on vibration isolators prevents vibrations from traveling through the floor and generating noise in areas where workers are present. Note that either the machine or the worker's area can be isolated.

REDUCE VIBRATING PARTS AND SURFACES
Panels rigidly connected to vibrating machinery can radiate more sound than the machine itself. Relocating instruments or control panels away from the vibrating machinery can help reduce the overall noise, and securing any loose parts can further decrease the noise level.

USE ANTI-VIBRATION CONNECTORS
Rigid connections can transfer vibrations to surfaces such as walls and ceilings, increasing radiated sound. Isolating these noise sources can help reduce the transmitted vibrations and decrease overall noise levels.

KEEP NOISY MACHINERY AWAY FROM WALLS
Sound reflects off hard surfaces such as walls, floors, and ceilings, which increases the overall noise levels in a space. Placing a noise source closer to a hard surface amplifies the reflected noise.

Generally, the optimal placement for a noise source is away from walls and suspended between the floor and ceiling. The least ideal placement is in corners, where sound will reflect off three surfaces, significantly increasing noise levels.

ADD SOUND ABSORPTION MATERIALS

Sound reflects easily off hard surfaces such as walls, ceilings, and floors, which increases noise levels within a space. Porous materials, such as textiles and foam, absorb sound. Covering hard surfaces with these absorptive materials helps reduce reflected sound and lowers overall noise levels.

Here are some best practices for using sound-absorbing materials:
- Use line enclosures, barriers, and screens with sound absorbers on the noisy side.
- Use thin materials to absorb high-frequency noise.
- Use thicker, absorptive materials to absorb lower-frequency noise.
- Hang sound-absorbent baffles so both sides are exposed to noise, maximizing surface area for absorption.
- Use hard perforated materials, such as stainless steel micro-perforated plates, in areas where barriers and enclosures require cleaning with high temperatures or pressure, such as cleanrooms and food production facilities.
- Consult vendors of sound-absorbing materials to help analyze noise levels and recommend commercially available products.

BUILD ENCLOSURES AROUND THE EQUIPMENT

Enclosures can effectively block the transmission of mid- and high-frequency sounds. Workplace tasks that commonly generate mid- to high-frequency noise include:
- riveting
- grinding operations
- machine cutting
- compressed air cleaning

INSTALL BARRIERS

High-frequency noise can be blocked using a barrier, also known as a "sound shield." The effectiveness of a barrier increases with its height and proximity to the noise source. Indoor barriers work best when the ceiling is sound-absorbent. While barriers are well-suited for high-frequency noise, they are generally less effective for low-frequency noise.

Workplace Noise | 59

Tips for Using Barriers between Noise Sources and Workers
- **Construct barriers from dense materials, such as brick or sheet steel.** Chipboard and plasterboard are also effective.
- **Place the barrier as close as possible to either the noise source or the worker's position.** Barriers in these locations block more sound than those placed halfway between.
- **Enhance ceilings with absorbent materials.** Add absorbent materials to ceilings to increase the effectiveness of indoor barriers.
- **Minimize reflections with sound-absorbing materials.** To eliminate reflections and reduce the overall sound level, cover the barrier with sound-absorbing material on the side facing the noise source.

SEAL ENCLOSURES FOR LOW-FREQUENCY SOURCES
Low-frequency noise can easily travel around corners, through openings, and spread in all directions, making barriers insufficient for effectively blocking it. To contain low-frequency noise, use a complete enclosure made of solid material lined with sound-absorbent material. Ensure that all doors and openings close tightly to maximize noise containment.

Tips for Enclosure Design
- Construct enclosures with dense material and line them with absorptive material for optimal sound reduction.
- Keep operator access openings as small as possible while maintaining usability.
- Use fully sealed enclosures to block low-frequency sound, as partial enclosures are not sufficient for this purpose.

Employers can greatly reduce workers' noise exposure by implementing engineering controls, such as modifying equipment, adding sound-absorbing materials, and designing enclosures effectively.[1]

---

[1] National Institute for Occupational Safety and Health (NIOSH) "Implement Engineering Controls," Centers for Disease Control and Prevention (CDC), February 16, 2024. Available online. URL: www.cdc.gov/niosh/noise/prevent/engineering.html. Accessed October 7, 2024.

Part 3 | Auditory Impairment: Diseases and Related Disorders

Chapter 7 | Infectious Diseases and Hearing Loss

Chapter Contents
Section 7.1—Ear Infections in Children 64
Section 7.2—Meningitis... 67
Section 7.3—Shingles 73

Section 7.1 | Ear Infections in Children

WHAT IS AN EAR INFECTION?

An ear infection is an inflammation of the middle ear, usually caused by bacteria, that occurs when fluid builds up behind the eardrum. Anyone can get an ear infection, but children get them more often than adults. Five out of six children will have at least one ear infection by their third birthday. In fact, ear infections are the most common reason parents bring their child to a doctor. The scientific name for an ear infection is "otitis media" (OM).

There are three main types of ear infections. Each has a different combination of symptoms.
1. **Acute otitis media (AOM).** It is the most common ear infection. Parts of the middle ear are infected and swollen, and fluid is trapped behind the eardrum. This causes pain in the ear—commonly called an "earache." Your child might also have a fever.
2. **Otitis media with effusion (OME).** This sometimes occurs after an ear infection has run its course, and fluid stays trapped behind the eardrum. A child with OME may have no symptoms, but a doctor can see the fluid behind the eardrum with a special instrument.
3. **Chronic otitis media with effusion (COME).** It occurs when fluid remains in the middle ear for a long time or returns repeatedly, even though there is no infection. COME makes it harder for children to fight new infections and can also affect their hearing.

HOW CAN I TELL IF MY CHILD HAS AN EAR INFECTION?

Most ear infections happen to children before they have learned how to talk. If your child is not old enough to say, "My ear hurts," here are a few things to look for:
- tugging or pulling at the ear(s)
- fussiness and crying
- trouble sleeping
- fever (especially in infants and younger children)

- fluid draining from the ear
- clumsiness or problems with balance
- trouble hearing or responding to quiet sounds

WHAT CAUSES AN EAR INFECTION?

An ear infection is usually caused by bacteria and often begins after a child has a sore throat, cold, or other upper respiratory infection. If the upper respiratory infection is bacterial, these same bacteria may spread to the middle ear; if the upper respiratory infection is caused by a virus, such as a cold, bacteria may be drawn to the microbe-friendly environment and move into the middle ear as a secondary infection. Because of the infection, fluid builds up behind the eardrum.

WHY ARE CHILDREN MORE LIKELY THAN ADULTS TO GET EAR INFECTIONS?

There are several reasons why children are more likely than adults to get ear infections.

Eustachian tubes are smaller and more level in children than they are in adults. This makes it difficult for fluid to drain out of the ear, even under normal conditions. If the Eustachian tubes are swollen or blocked with mucus due to a cold or other respiratory illness, fluid may not be able to drain.

A child's immune system is not as effective as an adult's because it is still developing. This makes it harder for children to fight infections.

As part of the immune system, the adenoids respond to bacteria passing through the nose and mouth. Sometimes bacteria get trapped in the adenoids, causing a chronic infection that can then pass on to the Eustachian tubes and the middle ear.

HOW DOES A DOCTOR DIAGNOSE A MIDDLE EAR INFECTION?

The first thing a doctor will do is ask about your child's health. Has your child had a head cold or sore throat recently? Is he having trouble sleeping? Is she pulling at her ears? If an ear infection seems likely, the simplest way for a doctor to tell is to use a lighted instrument called an "otoscope" to look at the eardrum. A red, bulging eardrum indicates an infection.

A doctor may also use a pneumatic otoscope, which blows a puff of air into the ear canal, to check for fluid behind the eardrum. A normal eardrum will move back and forth more easily than an eardrum with fluid behind it.

Tympanometry, which uses sound tones and air pressure, is a diagnostic test a doctor might use if the diagnosis is still unclear. A tympanometry device is a small, soft plug that contains a tiny microphone and speaker and varies air pressure in the ear. It measures how flexible the eardrum is at different pressures.

HOW IS AN ACUTE MIDDLE EAR INFECTION TREATED?

Many doctors will prescribe an antibiotic, such as amoxicillin, to be taken over 7–10 days. Your doctor may also recommend over-the-counter (OTC) pain relievers, such as acetaminophen or ibuprofen, or eardrops, to help with fever and pain. (Because aspirin is considered a major preventable risk factor for Reye syndrome, a child who has a fever or other flu-like symptoms should not be given aspirin unless instructed to do so by your doctor.)

If your doctor prescribes an antibiotic, it is important to make sure your child takes it exactly as prescribed and for the full amount of time. Even though your child may seem better in a few days, the infection still has not completely cleared from the ear. Stopping the medicine too soon could allow the infection to come back. It is also important to return for your child's follow-up visit so that the doctor can check if the infection is gone.

CAN EAR INFECTIONS BE PREVENTED?

Currently, the best way to prevent ear infections is to reduce the risk factors associated with them. Here are some things you might want to do to lower your child's risk for ear infections:

- **Vaccinate your child against the flu.** Make sure your child gets the influenza vaccine every year.
- **It is recommended that you vaccinate your child with the 13-valent pneumococcal conjugate vaccine (PCV13).** The PCV13 protects against more types of infection-causing bacteria than the previous vaccine, the PCV7. If your child has already begun PCV7 vaccination,

consult your physician about how to transition to PCV13. The Centers for Disease Control and Prevention (CDC) recommends that children under age two be vaccinated, starting at two months of age. Studies have shown that vaccinated children get far fewer ear infections than children who are not vaccinated. The vaccine is strongly recommended for children in daycare.
- **Wash hands frequently.** Washing hands prevents the spread of germs and can help keep your child from catching a cold or the flu.
- **Avoid exposing your baby to cigarette smoke.** Studies have shown that babies who are around smokers have more ear infections.
- **Never put your baby down for a nap or for the night with a bottle.**
- **Do not allow sick children to spend time together.** As much as possible, limit your child's exposure to other children when your child or your child's playmates are sick.[1]

Section 7.2 | Meningitis

WHAT IS MENINGITIS?

Meningitis is an infection of the membranes surrounding the brain and spinal cord, called the "meninges." It often appears with flu-like symptoms that develop over one to two days. Most cases of meningitis in the United States are caused by a viral infection, but it can also be caused by bacteria, parasites, and fungi.

The signs of meningitis may include:
- sudden fever
- severe headache
- nausea or vomiting

---

[1] "Ear Infections in Children," National Institute on Deafness and Other Communication Disorders (NIDCD), March 16, 2022. Available online. URL: www.nidcd.nih.gov/health/ear-infections-children. Accessed October 7, 2024.

- double vision
- sensitivity to bright light
- stiffness in the neck

Some forms of the disease typically involve distinctive rashes. Bacterial meningitis may be associated with kidney and adrenal gland failure and shock. Important signs to watch for in an infant include fever, lethargy, not waking for feedings, vomiting, body stiffness, unexplained or unusual irritability, and a full or bulging fontanel (the soft spot on the top of the head).

Some cases of meningitis improve on their own without treatment. Others require emergency treatment with antibiotics, which can cause death. Because the disease can occur suddenly and progress rapidly, anyone who is suspected of having meningitis should immediately contact a doctor or go to the hospital.

TYPES OF MENINGITIS

There are multiple kinds of meningitis, categorized by the cause of the infection or inflammation in the meninges.

Bacterial Meningitis

Bacterial meningitis is a rare but potentially fatal disease. Several types of bacteria can first cause an upper respiratory tract infection and then travel through the bloodstream to the brain. The disease can also occur when bacteria invade the meninges directly, rather than traveling from elsewhere in the body. Bacterial meningitis can cause stroke, hearing loss, and permanent brain damage. Types of bacterial meningitis are as follows:

- **Pneumococcal meningitis.** It is the most common and serious form of bacterial meningitis. It is caused by the bacteria *Streptococcus pneumoniae*, which also causes pneumonia, blood poisoning (septicemia), and ear and sinus infections. Pneumococcal meningitis is particularly dangerous for children under age two and adults with a weakened immune system. People who have had pneumococcal meningitis often suffer neurological damage, which can range from deafness to severe brain damage.

Vaccinations are available for some strains of the pneumococcal bacteria.
- **Meningococcal meningitis.** It is very contagious. It is caused by the bacteria *Neisseria meningitidis*. High-risk groups include infants, people with suppressed immune systems, travelers to foreign countries where the disease is common, and people who live in dormitories or barracks, including college students (freshmen in particular) and military recruits. Between 10 and 15 percent of cases of meningococcal meningitis are fatal, and another 10–15 percent cause brain damage and other serious side effects. People in close contact with a person diagnosed with meningococcal meningitis should be given preventative antibiotics.

Other forms of bacterial meningitis include the following:
- ***Listeria monocytogenes* meningitis.** It can sometimes spread through foods such as unpasteurized dairy or deli meats and is most common in older adults, newborns, and immunocompromised people.
- ***E. coli* meningitis.** It is more common in older adults, newborns, and individuals with implanted brain devices or who have had brain surgery. It may be transmitted from the parent to the baby through the birth canal.
- ***Mycobacterium tuberculosis* meningitis.** It is a rare disease that occurs when the bacteria that cause tuberculosis attack the meninges.
- ***Haemophilus influenzae* meningitis.** It was at one time the most common form of bacterial meningitis. Fortunately, the HIB (*Haemophilus influenzae* type b) vaccine has greatly reduced the number of cases in the United States. Those most at risk of getting this disease are children in child-care settings and children who do not have access to the vaccine.

Viral Meningitis
Viral meningitis is usually caused by enteroviruses. Enteroviruses are common viruses that usually enter the body through the mouth and

nose. Enteroviruses are present in mucus, saliva, and feces and can be transmitted through direct contact with an infected person or through contact with an infected object or surface. Other viruses that can cause meningitis include varicella zoster (the virus that causes chickenpox and shingles), influenza, mumps, HIV, and genital herpes.

Fungal Meningitis

Fungal infections can also cause meningitis. The most common form of fungal meningitis is caused by a fungus, *Cryptococcus neoformans*, found in bird droppings and dirt. Meningitis caused by this fungus (cryptococcal meningitis) mostly occurs in immunocompromised people but can also occur in healthy people. It can be slow to develop and live in the body for weeks before it shows symptoms. Although treatable, fungal meningitis often recurs in nearly half of affected individuals.

Parasites that cause meningitis are more common outside the United States and include cysticercosis (a tapeworm infection in the brain) and cerebral malaria. There are rare cases of meningitis caused by amoebas (single-cell organisms), sometimes related to freshwater swimming. These can be rapidly fatal.

WHO IS MORE LIKELY TO GET MENINGITIS?

Anyone can get meningitis. People with weakened immune systems, including people living with HIV/AIDS and those taking medications that suppress the activation of the immune system, are at increased risk.

Some forms of bacterial meningitis are contagious and can spread through contact with:
- saliva
- nasal discharge
- feces
- kissing, coughing, or sharing drinking glasses, eating utensils, or personal items such as toothbrushes

People sharing a household, at a daycare center, or in a classroom with an infected person can become infected. Any children who have not received routine vaccines are at increased risk of developing certain types of bacterial meningitis. Additional risk factors include recent travel and environmental exposure (such as being exposed to a parasite or bitten by an insect).

Not all meningitis is caused by infections. Non-infectious causes include autoimmune/rheumatological diseases and certain medications.

PREVENTING MENINGITIS

People should avoid sharing food, utensils, glasses, and other objects with someone who may be exposed to or have meningitis. All people should wash their hands often with soap and water. Communal living areas such as dormitories and barracks should be cleaned and sanitized regularly to avoid the spread of infections.

Effective vaccines are available to prevent *Haemophilus influenzae*, pneumococcal, and meningococcal meningitis.

People who live, work, or go to school with a person who has been diagnosed with bacterial meningitis may be prescribed antibiotics for a few days as a preventive measure.

To lessen the risk of being bitten by an infected mosquito or insect, people should take the following precautions:
- Limit outdoor activities at night.
- Wear pants and long-sleeved clothing when outdoors.
- Use insect repellents that are most effective for that particular region.
- Try to stay away from outdoor areas near freestanding pools of water where mosquitoes and other insects breed.

HOW IS MENINGITIS DIAGNOSED AND TREATED?
Diagnosing Meningitis

Early diagnosis of meningitis can make a big difference in a person's recovery or survival. Symptoms can appear suddenly and escalate to brain damage, hearing and/or vision loss, and even death. If a person is suspected of having meningitis, the healthcare provider will ask about activities conducted over the past several days or weeks, including travel, exposure to insects, contact with sick people, and so on. The doctor will also perform a physical exam and review the person's medical history to identify preexisting medical conditions and medications. Doctors may use various diagnostic tests to confirm the presence of infection or inflammation in the meninges.

Diagnostic tests for meningitis may include the following:
- **A neurological examination.** It involves a series of tests designed to assess movement and sensory function, nerve function, hearing and speech, vision, coordination and balance, mental status, and changes in mood or behavior.
- **Labs of blood, urine, and body secretions.** They can help detect and identify an infection in the brain or spinal cord and determine the presence of antibodies and foreign proteins. These tests can also rule out conditions that may have similar symptoms.
- **Analysis of the cerebrospinal fluid that surrounds and protects the brain and spinal cord.** It can detect infections, acute and chronic inflammation, and other diseases. Cerebrospinal fluid is obtained through a procedure called a "lumbar puncture."
- **Brain imaging.** It can reveal signs of inflammation, bleeding, or other abnormalities. A CT (computed tomography) or MRI (magnetic resonance imaging) scan can aid in diagnosing meningitis.

Treating Meningitis

People who are suspected of having meningitis should receive immediate, aggressive medical treatment. The disease can progress quickly and has the potential to cause severe, irreversible neurological damage.

Early treatment of bacterial meningitis involves antibiotics that can cross the blood-brain barrier. These antibiotics can greatly reduce the risk of dying from the disease. A doctor may also prescribe anticonvulsant medications to prevent seizures and corticosteroids (such as prednisone) to reduce brain inflammation, relieve pressure and swelling, and prevent hearing loss.

Antibiotics, developed to kill bacteria, are not effective against viruses. Fortunately, viral meningitis is rarely life-threatening, and no specific treatment is needed. Fungal meningitis is treated with intravenous antifungal medications.

Recovery

The outlook for individuals with meningitis generally depends on the type of meningitis, the severity of the illness, and how quickly treatment is given. In most cases, people with very mild meningitis can make a full recovery, although the process may be slow.

Individuals who experience only headache, fever, and stiff neck may recover in two to four weeks. Individuals with bacterial meningitis typically show some relief 48–72 hours following initial treatment but are more likely to experience complications of the disease.

In more serious cases, meningitis can cause hearing and/or speech loss, blindness, permanent brain and nerve damage, behavioral changes, cognitive disabilities, lack of muscle control, seizures, and memory loss. These individuals may need long-term therapy, medication, and supportive care.[1]

Section 7.3 | Shingles

WHAT IS SHINGLES?

Shingles, also called "herpes zoster," is a disease that triggers a painful skin rash. It is caused by the same virus as chickenpox, the varicella-zoster virus. After you recover from chickenpox (usually as a child), the virus continues to live in some of your nerve cells.

For most adults, the virus is inactive and does not lead to shingles. However, for about one in three adults, the virus will become active again and cause shingles.

WHAT ARE THE SYMPTOMS OF SHINGLES?

Usually, shingles develops on just one side of the body or face, and in a small area. The most common place for shingles to occur is in a band around one side of the waistline.

---

[1] "Meningitis," National Institute of Neurological Disorders and Stroke (NINDS), July 19, 2024. Available online. URL: www.ninds.nih.gov/health-information/disorders/meningitis. Accessed October 9, 2024.

Most people with shingles have one or more of the following symptoms:
- fluid-filled blisters
- burning, shooting pain
- tingling, itching, or numbness of the skin
- chills, fever, headache, or upset stomach

For some people, the symptoms of shingles are mild. They might just experience some itching. For others, shingles can cause intense pain that can be felt from the gentlest touch or breeze. It is important to talk with your doctor if you notice any shingles symptoms.

If you notice blisters on your face, see your doctor right away because this is an urgent problem. Blisters near or in the eye can cause lasting eye damage and blindness. Hearing loss, brief paralysis of the face, or, very rarely, inflammation of the brain (encephalitis) can also occur.

IS SHINGLES CONTAGIOUS?

If you are in contact with someone who has shingles, you will not get the symptoms of shingles yourself. However, direct contact with fluid from a shingles rash can still spread the varicella-zoster virus, which can cause chickenpox in people who have not had chickenpox before or the chickenpox vaccine. The risk of spreading the virus is low if the shingles rash is kept covered.

AM I AT RISK FOR SHINGLES?

Everyone who has had chickenpox is at risk of developing shingles. Researchers do not fully understand what makes the virus become active and cause shingles. However, certain factors make it more likely:
- **Older age.** The risk of developing shingles increases as you age. About half of all shingles cases occur in adults aged 60 or older. The chance of getting shingles becomes much greater by age 70.
- **Trouble fighting infections**. Your immune system is the part of your body that responds to infections. Age can affect your immune system. So can HIV, cancer, cancer

treatments, too much sun, and organ transplant drugs. Even stress or a cold can weaken your immune system for a short time. These factors can increase your risk for shingles.

Most people only have shingles one time. However, it is possible to have it more than once.

WHO SHOULD GET VACCINATED FOR SHINGLES?
Vaccination can significantly reduce the risk of developing shingles, especially in older adults. The current shingles vaccine (brand name Shingrix) is a safe, easy, and more effective way to prevent shingles than the previous vaccine. In fact, it is over 90 percent effective at preventing shingles. Most adults aged 50 and older should get vaccinated with the shingles vaccine, which is given in two doses. You can get the shingles vaccine at your doctor's office and at some pharmacies.

HOW LONG DOES SHINGLES LAST?
Most cases of shingles last three to five weeks.
- The initial symptom often includes a burning or tingling pain, sometimes accompanied by numbness or itching on one side of the body.
- One to five days later, a red rash typically appears at the site of discomfort.
- A few days following the rash, fluid-filled blisters develop.
- About one week to 10 days after that, the blisters dry up and crust over.
- A couple of weeks later, the scabs clear up.

In some cases, lingering pain, known as "postherpetic neuralgia," can persist for weeks, months, or even years after the rash has healed.
You should get the shingles vaccine if you:
- have already had chickenpox, the chickenpox vaccine, or shingles
- received the prior shingles vaccine called "Zostavax"
- do not remember having had chickenpox

Medicare Part D and private health insurance plans may cover some or all of the cost. Check with Medicare or your health plan to find out if it is covered.

You should not get vaccinated if you:
- currently have shingles
- are sick or have a fever
- had an allergic reaction to a previous dose of the shingles vaccine

If you are unsure about the above criteria or have other health concerns, talk with your doctor before getting the vaccine.

HOW IS SHINGLES DIAGNOSED AND TREATED?

If you think you might have shingles, talk to your doctor as soon as possible. It is important to see your doctor no later than three days after the rash starts. The doctor will confirm whether you have shingles and can make a treatment plan. Most cases can be diagnosed from a visual examination. If you have a condition that weakens the immune system, your doctor may order a shingles test. Although there is no cure for shingles, early treatment with antiviral medications can help the blisters clear up faster and limit severe pain. Shingles can often be treated at home.

TIPS FOR COPING WITH SHINGLES

If you have shingles, here are some tips that might help you feel better:
- Wear loose-fitting, natural-fiber clothing.
- Take an oatmeal bath or use calamine lotion to soothe your skin.
- Apply a cool washcloth to your blisters to ease the pain and help dry the blisters.
- Keep the area clean and try not to scratch the blisters so they do not become infected or leave a scar.
- Do things that take your mind off your pain. For example, watch TV, read, talk with friends, listen to relaxing music, or work on a hobby such as crafts or gardening.
- Get plenty of rest and eat well-balanced meals.

Infectious Diseases and Hearing Loss | 77

- Try simple exercises such as stretching or walking. Check with your doctor before starting a new exercise routine.
- Avoid stress, as it can make the pain worse.
- Share your feelings about your pain with family and friends and ask for their understanding.[1]

---

[1] National Institute on Aging (NIA), "Shingles," National Institutes of Health (NIH), October 12, 2021. Available online. URL: www.nia.nih.gov/health/shingles/shingles. Accessed October 9, 2024.

Chapter 8 | Congenital and Developmental Hearing Loss

Chapter Contents
Section 8.1—Congenital Cytomegalovirus and Its Effect on Hearing 80
Section 8.2—Enlarged Vestibular Aqueducts and Hearing Loss 82

Section 8.1 | Congenital Cytomegalovirus and Its Effect on Hearing

WHAT IS CYTOMEGALOVIRUS?

Cytomegalovirus (CMV) is a common virus that infects people of all ages. In the United States, nearly one in three children is already infected with CMV by age 5, and over half of adults have been infected with CMV by age 40.

Once CMV is in a person's body, it stays there for life and can reactivate. A person can also be re-infected with a different strain of the virus.

WHO IS AT RISK?

Anyone can get CMV. Some people are at higher risk for complications from CMV, such as those who are pregnant or have weakened immune systems.

If you are pregnant and infected with CMV, you can pass CMV to your developing baby. When a baby is born with a CMV infection, it is called "congenital CMV."

About 1 in 200 babies is born with congenital CMV infection. About one in five babies with congenital CMV infection will have birth defects or other long-term health problems.[1]

CONGENITAL CYTOMEGALOVIRUS AND HEARING LOSS

Hearing loss can occur at birth or later. Newborns with CMV may have hearing loss in one ear and may later develop hearing loss in the other ear. Hearing loss may progress from mild to severe during the first two years of life—a critical period for language learning.

Sometimes, hearing loss may worsen with age and progress through the teenage years. Over time, hearing loss can affect your child's ability to develop communication, language, and social skills.

---

[1] "About Cytomegalovirus," Centers for Disease Control and Prevention (CDC), May 30, 2024. Available online. URL: www.cdc.gov/cytomegalovirus/about/index.html. Accessed October 10, 2024.

Congenital and Developmental Hearing Loss | 81

SIGNS OF HEARING LOSS
In a Baby
- Does not startle at loud noises.
- Does not turn to the source of a sound after six months of age.
- Does not say single words, such as "dada" or "mama" by age one.
- Turns head when they see you but not if you only call out their name.
- Seems to hear some sounds but not others.

In a Child
- Speech is delayed.
- Speech is not clear.
- Does not follow directions (this could be the result of partial or complete hearing loss).
- Often says, "Huh?"
- Turns the TV volume up too high.

HEARING CHECKS AND THERAPIES
Babies with congenital CMV infection, with or without signs at birth, should have regular hearing checks.

SERVICES
Children diagnosed with hearing loss should receive services such as speech or occupational therapy. Children with hearing loss can also learn to communicate in other ways, like using:
- sign language
- devices such as hearing aids and cochlear implants

These services help ensure they develop important communication, language, and social skills. The earlier children with hearing loss start receiving services, the more likely they are to reach their full potential.

MEDICATION
Some babies with signs of congenital CMV at birth may benefit from medications called "antivirals."

Valganciclovir is an antiviral medication that might improve hearing and developmental outcomes. It can have serious side effects and has only been studied in babies with signs of congenital CMV infection. There is limited information on the effectiveness of valganciclovir to treat infants with hearing loss alone.

Babies who are treated with antivirals should be closely monitored by their doctor.[2]

Section 8.2 | Enlarged Vestibular Aqueducts and Hearing Loss

WHAT ARE VESTIBULAR AQUEDUCTS?

Vestibular aqueducts are narrow, bony canals that travel from the inner ear to deep inside the skull (see Figure 8.1). The aqueducts begin inside the temporal bone, the part of the skull just above the ear. The temporal bone also contains two sensory organs that are part of the inner ear. These organs are the cochlea, which detects sound waves and turns them into nerve signals, and the vestibular labyrinth, which detects movement and gravity. These organs, together with the nerves that send their signals to the brain, work to create normal hearing and balance. Running through each vestibular aqueduct is a fluid-filled tube called the "endolymphatic duct," which connects the inner ear to a balloon-shaped structure called the "endolymphatic sac."

Recent studies indicate that a vestibular aqueduct is abnormally enlarged if it is larger than 1 millimeter, roughly the size of the head of a pin. This is called an "enlarged vestibular aqueduct," or "EVA"; the condition is also known as a "dilated vestibular aqueduct" or a "large vestibular aqueduct." If a vestibular aqueduct is enlarged, the endolymphatic duct and sac usually grow

---

[2] "Congenital CMV and Hearing Loss," Centers for Disease Control and Prevention (CDC), May 10, 2024. Available online. URL: www.cdc.gov/cytomegalovirus/congenital-infection/hearing-loss.html. Accessed October 10, 2024.

Congenital and Developmental Hearing Loss | 83

large too. The functions of the endolymphatic duct and sac are not completely understood.

Scientists believe that the endolymphatic duct and sac help to ensure that the fluid in the inner ear contains the correct amounts of certain chemicals called "ions." Ions are needed to help start the nerve signals that send sound and balance information to the brain.

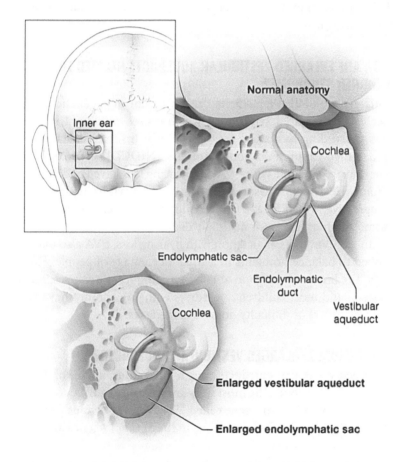

Figure 8.1. The Inner Ear
National Institutes of Health (NIH)

HOW ARE ENLARGED VESTIBULAR AQUEDUCTS RELATED TO CHILDHOOD HEARING LOSS?

Research suggests that most children with enlarged vestibular aqueducts (EVA) will develop some hearing loss. Scientists also find that 5–15 percent of children with sensorineural hearing loss (hearing loss caused by damage to sensory cells inside the cochlea) have EVA. However, scientists do not think that EVA causes hearing loss but that both are caused by the same underlying defect. EVA can be an important clue pointing to what is actually causing the hearing loss.

HOW ARE ENLARGED VESTIBULAR AQUEDUCTS RELATED TO PENDRED SYNDROME?

Enlarged vestibular aqueducts can be a sign of a genetic disorder called "Pendred syndrome," which causes childhood hearing loss. According to a study by the National Institute on Deafness and Other Communication Disorders (NIDCD), approximately one-fourth of people with EVA and hearing loss have Pendred syndrome. Hearing loss associated with Pendred syndrome is usually progressive, which means that a child will lose hearing over time. Some children may become totally deaf.

In addition to its association with hearing loss, EVA also may be linked to balance problems in a small percentage of people. However, the brain is very good at compensating for a weak vestibular system, and most children and adults with EVA do not have balance disorders or difficulty doing routine tasks.

WHAT CAUSES ENLARGED VESTIBULAR AQUEDUCTS?

Enlarged vestibular aqueducts have many causes, not all of which are fully understood. The most well-known cause of EVA and hearing loss is mutations in a gene called "*SLC26A4*" (previously known as the "PDS gene"). Two mutations in the *SLC26A4* gene can result in Pendred syndrome.

Scientists believe that other, currently unknown, genetic or environmental factors may also lead to EVA.

HOW ARE ENLARGED VESTIBULAR AQUEDUCTS DIAGNOSED?
Medical professionals use different clues to help them determine the cause of hearing loss. Two tests that are often used to identify the cause of hearing loss are magnetic resonance imaging (MRI) and computed tomography (CT) imaging of the inner ear. One or both tests are often recommended when evaluating a child with sensorineural hearing loss. This is particularly true when a child's hearing loss occurs suddenly, is greater in one ear than the other, or varies or gets worse over time. Although most CT scans of children with hearing loss are normal, EVA is the most commonly observed abnormality.

CAN ENLARGED VESTIBULAR AQUEDUCTS BE TREATED TO REDUCE HEARING LOSS?
No treatment has proven effective in reducing the hearing loss associated with EVA or in slowing its progression. Although some otolaryngologists (a doctor or surgeon who specializes in diseases of the ears, nose, throat, and head and neck) recommend steroids to treat sudden sensorineural hearing loss, there are no scientific studies to show that this is an effective treatment for EVA. In addition, surgery to drain liquid out of the endolymphatic duct and sac or to remove the endolymphatic duct and sac is not only ineffective in treating EVA, it can be harmful. Research has shown conclusively that these surgeries can destroy hearing.

To reduce the likelihood of progression of hearing loss, people with EVA should avoid contact sports that might lead to head injury; wear head protection when engaged in activities such as bicycle riding or skiing that might lead to head injury; and avoid situations that can lead to barotrauma (extreme, rapid changes in air pressure), such as scuba diving or hyperbaric oxygen treatment. The pressure changes associated with flying in airplanes have also been reported to cause hearing loss in people with EVA. However, this is a rare event in commercial aircraft with pressurized cabins. If you have EVA, you can minimize your risk of hearing loss associated with air travel by taking nasal decongestants if you have sinus or nasal congestion, such as during a cold or flu.

Identifying hearing loss as early as possible is the best way to reduce EVA's effect. The earlier hearing loss is identified in children, the sooner they can develop skills that will help them learn and communicate with others. Children with permanent and progressive hearing loss, which is often linked with EVA, will benefit from learning other forms of communication, such as sign language or cued speech, or using assistive devices, such as a hearing aid or cochlear implant.[1]

---

[1] "Enlarged Vestibular Aqueducts and Childhood Hearing Loss," National Institute on Deafness and Other Communication Disorders (NIDCD), February 13, 2017. Available online. URL: www.nidcd.nih.gov/health/enlarged-vestibular-aqueducts-and-childhood-hearing-loss. Accessed October 7, 2024.

Chapter 9 | Chronic and Acquired Disorders

Chapter Contents
Section 9.1—Ménière Disease 88
Section 9.2—Tinnitus 90
Section 9.3—Otosclerosis.. 96
Section 9.4—Balance Disorders.. 97
Section 9.5—Auditory Neuropathy..................................... 103
Section 9.6—Sudden Deafness... 106
Section 9.7—Hearing Problems as a Late Effect of Childhood
 Cancer Treatment 109
Section 9.8—Congenital Zika Syndrome............................... 111

Section 9.1 | Ménière Disease

WHAT IS MÉNIÈRE DISEASE?

Ménière disease is a disorder of the inner ear that causes severe dizziness (vertigo), ringing in the ears (tinnitus), hearing loss, and a feeling of fullness or congestion in the ear. Ménière disease usually affects only one ear, but in 15–25 percent of people with the disorder, both ears may be affected.

Attacks of dizziness may come on suddenly or after a short period of tinnitus or muffled hearing. Some people have single attacks of dizziness separated by long periods of time. Others may experience many attacks close together over several days. Some people with Ménière disease have vertigo so extreme that they lose their balance and fall. These episodes are called "drop attacks."

Ménière disease is rare in children younger than 18. According to the American Academy of Otolaryngology-Head and Neck Surgery, Ménière disease can develop at any age, but it is more likely to occur in adults between 40 and 60 years of age. Approximately, 615,000 individuals in the United States have Ménière disease, and about 45,500 cases are newly diagnosed each year, according to the American Hearing Research Foundation.

WHAT CAUSES MÉNIÈRE DISEASE?

Theories vary about the causes of Ménière disease. Some researchers believe it may develop from constricted blood vessels, which also occur with migraine headaches. Other theories suggest viral infections, allergies, or autoimmune reactions as possible causes. Genetic variations could also play a role since Ménière disease sometimes affects more than one family member.

HOW IS MÉNIÈRE DISEASE DIAGNOSED?

Ménière disease is most often diagnosed and treated by an otolaryngologist (commonly called an "ear, nose, and throat doctor," or "ENT"). There is no definitive test or single symptom that a doctor can use to make a diagnosis. Your doctor may suggest a hearing screening to identify any hearing loss. To rule out other diseases, magnetic resonance imaging (MRI) or computed tomography (CT) scans of the brain may be recommended.

A diagnosis of definite Ménière disease is based on your medical history and the presence of:
- two or more spontaneous episodes of vertigo lasting 20 minutes to 12 hours
- hearing loss in one or both ears for low- to medium-frequency sounds, documented by a hearing test before, during, or after one of the episodes of vertigo
- hearing-related symptoms that occur irregularly; for example, tinnitus, hearing loss, or a feeling of fullness in the affected ear
- symptoms not accounted for by another diagnosed balance-related condition

Probable Ménière disease is typically diagnosed when you have all the symptoms listed above except hearing loss confirmed by a hearing test before, during, or after an episode of vertigo.

HOW IS MÉNIÈRE DISEASE TREATED?

There is not a cure yet for Ménière disease, and because symptoms can vary widely, the benefit of treatment options can be hard to gauge. Your doctor may recommend one or more of these management options to help you cope with your symptoms:
- **Dietary and behavioral changes.** Limiting dietary salt to 1,500–2,000 milligrams per day and taking a diuretic (water pill) may help control symptoms of Ménière disease. Quitting smoking may also reduce symptoms.
- **Medications.** The most disabling symptom of a Ménière disease attack is dizziness. Prescription drugs can help relieve dizziness and shorten the attack, particularly when taken soon after it starts.
- **Vestibular rehabilitation/physical therapy.** A doctor may recommend vestibular rehabilitation and/or physical therapy if you have chronic balance issues.
- **Injections.** Injecting the antibiotic gentamicin into the middle ear helps to control vertigo but significantly raises

the risk of hearing loss because gentamicin can damage the microscopic hair cells in the inner ear that help us hear. Corticosteroid injections are an alternative because they often reduce dizziness and have little to no risk of hearing loss.
- **Surgery.** Surgery may be recommended when all other treatments have failed to relieve dizziness. One surgical procedure decompresses the endolymphatic sac. Another surgical approach, used less frequently, cuts the vestibular nerve.

Although scientists have studied alternative therapies for Ménière disease, there is no evidence to show their effectiveness. This includes acupuncture, acupressure, tai chi, and herbal supplements, including ginkgo biloba, niacin, and ginger root. Be sure to tell your doctor if you are using alternative therapies since they can sometimes influence the effectiveness or safety of conventional medicines.

If you have hearing loss associated with Ménière disease, consider discussing hearing aid options with your doctor (www.nidcd.nih.gov/health/hearing-aids).[1]

Section 9.2 | Tinnitus

WHAT IS TINNITUS?

Tinnitus is the perception of sound that does not have an external source, so other people cannot hear it.

Tinnitus is commonly described as a ringing sound, but some people hear other types of sounds, such as roaring or buzzing. Tinnitus is common, with surveys estimating that 10–25 percent of adults have it. Children can also have tinnitus. For children and adults, tinnitus may improve or even go away over time, but in some

---

[1] "Ménière's Disease," National Institute on Deafness and Other Communication Disorders (NIDCD), August 15, 2024. Available online. URL: www.nidcd.nih.gov/health/menieres-disease. Accessed October 9, 2024.

cases, it worsens with time. When tinnitus lasts for three months or longer, it is considered chronic.

The causes of tinnitus are unclear, but most people who have it have some degree of hearing loss. Tinnitus is only rarely associated with a serious medical problem and is usually not severe enough to interfere with daily life. However, some people find that it affects their mood and their ability to sleep or concentrate. In severe cases, tinnitus can lead to anxiety or depression.

Currently, there is no cure for tinnitus, but there are ways to reduce symptoms. Common approaches include the use of sound therapy devices (including hearing aids), behavioral therapies, and medications.

WHAT ARE THE SYMPTOMS OF TINNITUS?

The symptoms of tinnitus can vary significantly from person to person. You may hear phantom sounds in one ear, in both ears, or in your head. The phantom sound may ring, buzz, roar, whistle, hum, click, hiss, or squeal. The sound may be soft or loud and may be low or high pitched. It may come and go or be present all the time. Sometimes, moving your head, neck, or eyes, or touching certain parts of your body may produce tinnitus symptoms or temporarily change the quality of the perceived sound. This is called "somatosensory tinnitus."

Most cases of tinnitus are subjective, meaning that only you can hear the sounds. In rare cases, the sound pulsates rhythmically, often in time with your heartbeat. In these cases, a doctor may be able to hear the sounds with a stethoscope, and if so, it is considered to be "objective tinnitus." Often, objective tinnitus has an identifiable cause and is treatable.

WHAT CAUSES TINNITUS?

While the exact causes of tinnitus are not fully understood, it has been linked to the following:
- **Noise exposure**. Many people experience tinnitus after being exposed to loud noise in a workplace setting or at a sporting event or concert. Tinnitus is also the most common service-related disability among veterans because

of loud noise they may have experienced from gunfire, machinery, bomb blasts, or other similar sources.
- **Hearing loss**. This can be caused by factors such as aging or exposure to loud noises, is strongly associated with tinnitus. Some people with hearing loss, however, never develop tinnitus.
- **Medications**. Tinnitus can be a side effect of taking certain medications, especially if they are taken at high doses. Medications associated with tinnitus include non-steroidal anti-inflammatory drugs (e.g., ibuprofen, naproxen, and aspirin), certain antibiotics, anti-cancer drugs, anti-malaria medications, and antidepressants.
- **Earwax or an ear infection**. Blockage of the ear canal by earwax or by fluid from an ear infection can trigger tinnitus.
- **Head or neck injuries**. A head or neck injury can damage structures of the ear, the nerve that carries sound signals to the brain, or areas of the brain that process sound, causing tinnitus.

Less common tinnitus risk factors include:
- **Ménière disease**. Tinnitus can be a symptom of Ménière disease, an inner ear disorder that can also cause balance problems and hearing loss.
- **Jaw joint problems**. The joint that connects the lower jaw to the skull is close to the ear. Jaw clenching or tooth grinding can damage surrounding tissue, causing or worsening tinnitus.
- **Tumor-related disorders**. A vestibular schwannoma (acoustic neuroma) is a benign tumor on a nerve that leads from the inner ear to the brain. Acoustic neuromas and other head, neck, and brain tumors can cause tinnitus.
- **Blood vessel problems**. High blood pressure (HBP), atherosclerosis, or malformations in blood vessels, especially if they are in or close to the ear, can alter blood flow and cause tinnitus.

- **Chronic conditions**. Diabetes, migraines, thyroid disorders, anemia, and certain autoimmune disorders such as lupus and multiple sclerosis are among the chronic conditions that have been linked to tinnitus.

While there are many possible causes of tinnitus, some people develop it for no known reason.

WHAT CREATES THE PERCEPTION OF NOISE IN THE EARS?

One leading theory is that tinnitus can occur when damage to the inner ear changes the signal carried by nerves to the parts of the brain that process sound. While tinnitus may seem to occur in your ear, the phantom sounds are instead generated by your brain, in an area called the "auditory cortex."

Other evidence shows that abnormal interactions between the auditory cortex and other neural circuits may play a role in tinnitus. The auditory cortex communicates with other parts of the brain, such as the parts that control attention and emotions, and studies have shown that some people with tinnitus have changes in these nonauditory brain regions.

HOW IS TINNITUS DIAGNOSED?

If you have tinnitus, first see your primary care doctor. Your doctor will check for earwax or fluid from an ear infection that could be blocking your ear canal. Your doctor will also ask about your medical history to determine whether an underlying condition or medication may be causing your tinnitus.

Next, you may be referred to an otolaryngologist (commonly called an "ear, nose, and throat doctor," or "ENT"). The ENT will ask you to describe the tinnitus sounds and when they started and will examine your head, neck, and ears. You might also be referred to an audiologist, who can measure your hearing and evaluate your tinnitus.

The ENT may order imaging tests, especially if your tinnitus pulsates. Imaging tests such as magnetic resonance imaging (MRI), computed tomography (CT), or ultrasound can help reveal whether a structural problem or underlying medical condition is causing your tinnitus.

WHAT TREATMENTS CAN HELP TINNITUS?

When tinnitus has an underlying physiological cause, such as earwax or jaw joint problems, addressing the cause can eliminate or greatly reduce symptoms. But for many people, symptoms can persist for months or even years. There are several ways to lessen the effect of tinnitus. Below are some of the treatments that your doctor may recommend.

- **Sound therapies.** These therapies are based partly on the view that tinnitus stems from changes in neural circuits in the brain brought on by hearing loss. Some evidence suggests that exposure to sound can reverse some of these neural changes and help silence tinnitus. Sound therapy may also work by masking the tinnitus sounds, helping you grow accustomed to them, or distracting you. Several types of devices are used in sound therapy. They include the following:
    - **Tabletop or smartphone sound generators are typically used as an aid for relaxation or sleep.** Placed near your bed, you can program a generator or set up a smartphone app to play pleasant sounds such as waves, waterfalls, rain, or the sounds of a summer night. You may also use other sound generators, such as a radio or a household fan. If your tinnitus is mild, this might be all that you need to help you fall asleep.
    - **Hearing aids are one of the main treatment options for people with tinnitus who have hearing loss.** They amplify external noises, allowing you to better engage with the world while also making your tinnitus less noticeable.
    - **Wearable sound generators are small electronic devices that fit in the ear like hearing aids and emit soft, pleasant sounds.** Because they are portable, they can provide continuous relief from tinnitus throughout the day. Smartphone apps may also be used to generate these sounds.
    - **Combination devices, which fit into the ear like hearing aids, provide sound amplification and

sound generation in one device. These devices are another option for treating tinnitus in people with hearing loss.
- **Behavioral therapy.** Counseling can improve your well-being by helping you reduce the effect of tinnitus on your life.
  - **Education about tinnitus can reduce anxiety by helping you recognize that the condition, in most cases, is unlikely to be linked to a serious medical condition.** Through counseling, you can learn coping techniques and strategies to avoid making symptoms worse, such as by limiting your exposure to loud noise.
  - **Cognitive-behavioral therapy (CBT) teaches you how to identify negative thoughts that cause you distress.** Your counselor will train you to change your response to negative thoughts and to focus on positive changes you can make to reduce the effect of tinnitus on your life. Studies have shown that this type of therapy can help improve the well-being of people with the condition.
  - **Tinnitus retraining therapy uses counseling and sound therapy to "retrain" the brain, both emotionally and physiologically, so that you no longer notice your tinnitus.** The counseling aspect of therapy aims to help you reclassify tinnitus sounds as neutral, while the continuous low-level sound from a device worn in the ear helps you get used to the presence of tinnitus.
- **Medications.** No medications specifically treat tinnitus, but your doctor may prescribe antidepressants or anti-anxiety medications to improve your mood or help you sleep. While certain vitamins, herbal extracts, and dietary supplements are commonly advertised as cures for the condition, none of these has been proven to be effective.[1]

---

[1] "Tinnitus," National Institute on Deafness and Other Communication Disorders (NIDCD), May 1, 2023. Available online. URL: www.nidcd.nih.gov/health/tinnitus. Accessed October 9, 2024.

Section 9.3 | Otosclerosis

WHAT IS OTOSCLEROSIS?

Otosclerosis is a term derived from "oto," meaning "of the ear," and "sclerosis," meaning "abnormal hardening of body tissue." The condition is caused by abnormal bone remodeling in the middle ear. Bone remodeling is a lifelong process in which bone tissue renews itself by replacing old tissue with new. In otosclerosis, abnormal remodeling disrupts the ability of sound to travel from the middle ear to the inner ear. Otosclerosis affects more than 3 million Americans. Many cases of otosclerosis are thought to be inherited. White, middle-aged women are most at risk.

WHAT CAUSES OTOSCLEROSIS?

Otosclerosis is most often caused when the stapes bone in the middle ear becomes stuck in place. When this bone is unable to vibrate, sound cannot travel through the ear, and hearing becomes impaired.

Why this happens is still unclear, but scientists think it could be related to a previous measles infection, stress fractures to the bony tissue surrounding the inner ear, or immune disorders. Otosclerosis also tends to run in families.

It may also have to do with the interaction among three different immune-system cells known as "cytokines." Researchers believe that the proper balance of these three substances is necessary for healthy bone remodeling and that an imbalance in their levels could cause the kind of abnormal remodeling that occurs in otosclerosis.

WHAT ARE THE SYMPTOMS OF OTOSCLEROSIS?

Hearing loss—the most frequently reported symptom of otosclerosis—usually starts in one ear and then moves to the other. This loss may appear very gradually. Many people with otosclerosis first notice that they are unable to hear low-pitched sounds or cannot hear a whisper. Some people may also experience dizziness, balance problems, or tinnitus. Tinnitus is a ringing, roaring, buzzing, or hissing in the ears or head that sometimes occurs with hearing loss.

HOW IS OTOSCLEROSIS DIAGNOSED?

Otosclerosis is diagnosed by health-care providers who specialize in hearing. These include an otolaryngologist (commonly called an "ear, nose, and throat doctor," or "ENT") because they are doctors who specialize in diseases of the ears, nose, throat, and neck); an otologist (a doctor who specializes in diseases of the ears); or an audiologist (a health-care professional trained to identify, measure, and treat hearing disorders). The first step in a diagnosis is to rule out other diseases or health problems that can cause the same symptoms as otosclerosis. Next steps include hearing tests that measure hearing sensitivity (audiogram) and middle-ear sound conduction (tympanogram). Sometimes, imaging tests—such as a CT scan—are also used to diagnose otosclerosis.

HOW IS OTOSCLEROSIS TREATED?

Currently, there is no effective drug treatment for otosclerosis, although there is hope that continued bone-remodeling research could identify potential new therapies. Mild otosclerosis can be treated with a hearing aid that amplifies sound, but surgery is often required. In a procedure known as a "stapedectomy," a surgeon inserts a prosthetic device into the middle ear to bypass the abnormal bone, permit sound waves to travel to the inner ear, and restore hearing.

It is important to discuss any surgical procedure with an ear specialist to clarify potential risks and limitations of the operation. For example, some hearing loss may persist after stapedectomy, and in rare cases, surgery can actually worsen hearing loss.[1]

Section 9.4 | Balance Disorders

WHAT IS A BALANCE DISORDER?

A balance disorder is a condition that makes one feel unsteady or dizzy. Whether standing, sitting, or lying down, a person might feel

---

[1] "Otosclerosis," National Institute on Deafness and Other Communication Disorders (NIDCD), March 16, 2022. Available online. URL: www.nidcd.nih.gov/health/otosclerosis. Accessed October 9, 2024.

as if they are moving, spinning, or floating. While walking, one might suddenly feel as if they are tipping over.

Everyone experiences a dizzy spell now and then, but the term "dizziness" can mean different things to different people. For one person, dizziness might mean a fleeting feeling of faintness, while for another, it could be an intense sensation of spinning (vertigo) that lasts a long time.

About 15 percent of American adults (33 million) had a balance or dizziness problem in 2008. Balance disorders can be caused by certain health conditions, medications, or problems in the inner ear or the brain. They can profoundly affect daily activities and cause psychological and emotional hardship.

WHAT ARE THE SYMPTOMS OF A BALANCE DISORDER?

If one has a balance disorder, symptoms might include:
- dizziness or vertigo (a spinning sensation)
- falling or feeling as if one is going to fall
- staggering when trying to walk
- lightheadedness, faintness, or a floating sensation
- blurred vision
- confusion or disorientation

Other symptoms might include:
- nausea and vomiting
- diarrhea
- changes in heart rate and blood pressure
- fear, anxiety, or panic

Symptoms may come and go over short time periods or last for a long time and can lead to fatigue and depression.

WHAT CAUSES BALANCE DISORDERS?

Balance problems can be caused by medications, ear infections, head injuries, or anything else that affects the inner ear or brain. Low blood pressure can lead to dizziness when one stands up too quickly. Problems that affect the skeletal or visual systems, such as arthritis or eye muscle imbalance, can also cause balance disorders. The risk of having balance problems increases with age.

Unfortunately, many balance disorders start suddenly and with no obvious cause.

HOW DOES MY BODY KEEP ITS BALANCE?

The sense of balance relies on a series of signals to the brain from several organs and structures in the body, specifically the eyes, ears, and the muscles and touch sensors in the legs. The part of the ear that assists in balance is known as the "vestibular system," or the "labyrinth," a maze-like structure in the inner ear made of bone and soft tissue.

Within the labyrinth are structures known as "semicircular canals." The semicircular canals contain three fluid-filled ducts, which form loops arranged roughly at right angles to one another. They inform the brain when the head rotates. Inside each canal is a gelatin-like structure called the "cupula," stretched like a thick sail that blocks off one end of each canal. The cupula sits on a cluster of sensory hair cells. Each hair cell has tiny, thin extensions called "stereocilia" that protrude into the cupula.

When one turns their head, fluid inside the semicircular canals moves, causing the cupulae to flex or billow like sails in the wind. This bends the stereocilia, creating a nerve signal sent to the brain to indicate which way the head has turned.

Between the semicircular canals and the cochlea (a snail-shaped, fluid-filled structure in the inner ear) lie two otolithic organs: fluid-filled pouches called the "utricle" and the "saccule." These organs inform the brain of the position of the head with respect to gravity, such as whether one is sitting up, leaning back, or lying down, as well as any direction the head might be moving, such as side to side, up or down, or forward or backward.

The utricle and the saccule also have sensory hair cells lining the floor or wall of each organ, with stereocilia extending into an overlying gel-like layer. Here, the gel contains tiny, dense grains of calcium carbonate called "otoconia." Regardless of the position of the head, gravity pulls on these grains, which then move the stereocilia to signal the head's position to the brain. Any head movement creates a signal that informs the brain about the change in head position.

When one moves, the vestibular system detects mechanical forces, including gravity, that stimulate the semicircular canals and the otolithic organs. These organs work with other sensory systems in the body, such as vision and the musculoskeletal sensory system, to control the position of the body at rest or in motion. This helps maintain a stable posture and keep balance when walking or running. It also aids in maintaining a stable visual focus on objects when the body changes position.

When the signals from any of these sensory systems malfunction, one can experience problems with their sense of balance, including dizziness or vertigo. If there are additional problems with motor control, such as weakness, slowness, tremor, or rigidity, the ability to recover properly from imbalance can be compromised. This raises the risk of falling and injury.

WHAT ARE SOME TYPES OF BALANCE DISORDERS?

There are more than a dozen different balance disorders. Some of the most common are:

- **Benign paroxysmal positional vertigo (BPPV) or positional vertigo.** A brief, intense episode of vertigo triggered by a specific change in the position of the head. One might feel as if they are spinning when bending down to look under something, tilting their head to look up or over their shoulder, or rolling over in bed. BPPV occurs when loose otoconia tumble into one of the semicircular canals and affect how the cupula works. This keeps the cupula from flexing properly, sending incorrect information about the head's position to the brain and causing vertigo. BPPV can result from a head injury or can develop just from aging.
- **Labyrinthitis.** An infection or inflammation of the inner ear that causes dizziness and loss of balance. It is often associated with an upper respiratory infection, such as the flu.
- **Ménière disease.** Episodes of vertigo, hearing loss, tinnitus (a ringing or buzzing in the ear), and a feeling of fullness in the ear. It may be associated with a change in

fluid volume within parts of the labyrinth, but the cause or causes remain unknown.
- **Vestibular neuronitis.** An inflammation of the vestibular nerve that can be caused by a virus and primarily causes vertigo.
- **Perilymph fistula.** A leakage of inner ear fluid into the middle ear. It causes unsteadiness that usually increases with activity, along with dizziness and nausea. Perilymph fistula can occur after a head injury, dramatic changes in air pressure (such as when scuba diving), physical exertion, ear surgery, or chronic ear infections. Some people are born with perilymph fistula.
- **Mal de Débarquement syndrome (MdDS).** A feeling of continuously rocking, swaying, or bobbing, typically after an ocean cruise or other sea travel, or even after prolonged running on a treadmill. Usually, the symptoms go away within a few hours or days after reaching land or stopping the treadmill. Severe cases, however, can last months or even years, and the cause remains unknown.

HOW ARE BALANCE DISORDERS DIAGNOSED?

Diagnosis of a balance disorder can be difficult. To determine if one has a balance problem, a primary doctor may suggest seeing an otolaryngologist and an audiologist. An otolaryngologist is a physician and surgeon who specializes in diseases and disorders of the ear, nose, neck, and throat. An audiologist is a clinician who specializes in the function of the hearing and vestibular systems.

One may be asked to participate in a hearing examination, blood tests, a video nystagmogram (a test that measures eye movements and the muscles that control them), or imaging studies of the head and brain. Another possible test is called "posturography." For this test, one stands on a special movable platform in front of a patterned screen.

Posturography measures how well one can maintain a steady balance during different platform conditions, such as standing on an unfixed, movable surface. Other tests, such as rotational chair testing, brisk head-shaking testing, or even tests that measure eye or neck muscle responses to brief clicks of sound, may also be performed. The vestibular system is complex, so multiple tests may be needed to best evaluate the cause of the balance problem.

HOW ARE BALANCE DISORDERS TREATED?

The first thing an otolaryngologist will do if one has a balance problem is determine if another health condition or a medication is to blame. If so, the doctor will treat the condition, suggest a different medication, or refer one to a specialist if the condition is outside their expertise.

If diagnosed with BPPV, the otolaryngologist or audiologist might perform a series of simple movements, such as the "Epley maneuver," to help dislodge the otoconia from the semicircular canal. In many cases, one session works; other people need the procedure several times to relieve their dizziness.

If diagnosed with Ménière disease, the otolaryngologist may recommend making some changes to one's diet and, if a smoker, that they stop smoking. Anti-vertigo or anti-nausea medications may relieve symptoms, but they can also cause drowsiness. Other medications, such as gentamicin (an antibiotic) or corticosteroids, may be used. Although gentamicin may reduce dizziness better than corticosteroids, it occasionally causes permanent hearing loss. In some severe cases of Ménière disease, surgery on the vestibular organs may be needed.

Some people with a balance disorder may not be able to fully relieve their dizziness and will need to find ways to cope with it. A vestibular rehabilitation therapist can help develop an individualized treatment plan.

One should talk to their doctor about whether it is safe to drive and about ways to lower the risk of falling and getting hurt during daily activities, such as walking up or down stairs, using the bathroom, or exercising. To reduce the risk of injury from dizziness, avoid walking in the dark. Wear low-heeled shoes or walking shoes outdoors. If necessary, use a cane or walker and modify conditions at home and in the workplace, such as adding handrails.[1]

---

[1] "Balance Disorders," National Institute on Deafness and Other Communication Disorders (NIDCD), March 6, 2018. Available online. URL: www.nidcd.nih.gov/health/balance-disorders. Accessed October 9, 2024.

Section 9.5 | Auditory Neuropathy

WHAT IS AUDITORY NEUROPATHY?

Auditory neuropathy is a hearing disorder in which the inner ear successfully detects sound but has a problem with sending sound from the ear to the brain. It can affect people of all ages, from infancy through adulthood. The number of people affected by auditory neuropathy is not known, but current information suggests that auditory neuropathies play a substantial role in hearing impairments and deafness.

When their hearing sensitivity is tested, people with auditory neuropathy may have normal hearing or hearing loss ranging from mild to severe. They always have poor speech-perception abilities, meaning that they have trouble understanding speech clearly. People with auditory neuropathy experience greater impairment in speech perception than hearing health experts would predict based on their degree of hearing loss on a hearing test. For example, a person with auditory neuropathy may be able to hear sounds but would still have difficulty recognizing spoken words. Sounds may fade in and out or seem out of sync for these individuals.

WHAT CAUSES AUDITORY NEUROPATHY?

Researchers report several causes of auditory neuropathy. In some cases, the cause may involve damage to the inner hair cells—specialized sensory cells in the inner ear that transmit information about sounds through the nervous system to the brain. In other cases, the cause may involve damage to the auditory neurons that transmit sound information from the inner hair cells to the brain. Other possible causes may include inheriting genes with mutations or suffering damage to the auditory system, either of which may result in faulty connections between the inner hair cells and the auditory nerve (the nerve leading from the inner ear to the brain) or damage to the auditory nerve itself. A combination of these problems may occur in some cases.

WHAT ARE THE ROLES OF THE OUTER AND INNER HAIR CELLS?

Outer hair cells help amplify sound vibrations entering the inner ear from the middle ear. When hearing is functioning normally, the inner hair cells convert these vibrations into electrical signals that travel as nerve impulses to the brain, where the brain interprets the impulses as sound.

Although outer hair cells—cells next to and more numerous than inner hair cells—are generally more prone to damage than inner hair cells, outer hair cells seem to function normally in people with auditory neuropathy.

ARE THERE RISK FACTORS FOR AUDITORY NEUROPATHY?

There are several ways that children may acquire auditory neuropathy. Some children diagnosed with auditory neuropathy experienced particular health problems before or during birth or as newborns. These problems include inadequate oxygen supply during or prior to birth, premature birth, jaundice, low birth weight, and dietary thiamine deficiency. In addition, some drugs used to treat pregnant women or newborns may damage the baby's inner hair cells, causing auditory neuropathy. Adults may also develop auditory neuropathy along with age-related hearing loss.

Auditory neuropathy runs in some families, and in some cases, scientists have identified genes with mutations that compromise the ear's ability to transmit sound information to the brain. Thus, the inheritance of mutated genes is also a risk factor for auditory neuropathy.

Some people with auditory neuropathy have neurological disorders that also cause problems outside of the hearing system. Examples of such disorders include Charcot-Marie-Tooth syndrome and Friedreich ataxia.

HOW IS AUDITORY NEUROPATHY DIAGNOSED?

Health professionals—including otolaryngologists (ear, nose, and throat (ENT) doctors), pediatricians, and audiologists—use a combination of methods to diagnose auditory neuropathy. These include tests of auditory brainstem response (ABR) and otoacoustic emissions (OAE). The hallmark of auditory neuropathy is an absent or highly abnormal ABR reading together with a normal OAE reading. A normal OAE reading is a sign that the outer hair cells are functioning appropriately.

An ABR test uses electrodes placed on a person's head and ears to monitor brain wave activity in response to sound. An OAE test uses a small, very sensitive microphone inserted into the ear canal to monitor the faint sounds produced by the outer hair cells in response to auditory stimulation. ABR and OAE testing are painless and can be used for newborn babies and infants as well as older children and adults. Other tests may also be used as part of a comprehensive evaluation of an individual's hearing and speech-perception abilities.

DOES AUDITORY NEUROPATHY EVER GET BETTER OR WORSE?

Some newborn babies diagnosed with auditory neuropathy improve and start to hear and speak within a year or two. Other infants remain the same, while some worsen and show signs that the outer hair cells no longer function (abnormal otoacoustic emissions). Depending on the underlying cause, hearing sensitivity can remain stable, improve, or gradually worsen in people with auditory neuropathy.

WHAT TREATMENTS, DEVICES, AND OTHER APPROACHES CAN HELP PEOPLE WITH AUDITORY NEUROPATHY TO COMMUNICATE?

Researchers are still seeking effective treatments for people with auditory neuropathy. Meanwhile, professionals in the hearing field differ in their opinions about the potential benefits of hearing aids, cochlear implants, and other technologies for people with auditory neuropathy. Some professionals report that hearing aids and personal listening devices, such as frequency modulation (FM) systems, are helpful for some children and adults with auditory neuropathy. Cochlear implants (electronic devices that compensate for damaged or nonworking parts of the inner ear) may also help some people with auditory neuropathy. No tests are currently available, however, to determine whether an individual with auditory neuropathy might benefit from a hearing aid or cochlear implant.

Debate also continues about the best ways to educate and improve communication skills in infants and children who have hearing impairments, such as auditory neuropathy. One approach favors sign language as the child's first language. A second approach encourages the use of listening skills—together with technologies such as hearing aids and cochlear implants—and spoken language. A combination of these two approaches may also be used. Some health professionals believe it may be especially difficult for children with auditory neuropathy to learn to communicate only through spoken language because their ability to understand speech is often severely impaired. Adults with auditory neuropathy and older children who have already developed spoken language may benefit from learning how to speech-read (also known as "lipreading").[1]

Section 9.6 | Sudden Deafness

WHAT IS SUDDEN DEAFNESS?

Sudden sensorineural (inner ear) hearing loss (SSHL), commonly known as "sudden deafness," is an unexplained, rapid loss of hearing that occurs either all at once or over a few days. SSHL occurs because something is wrong with the sensory organs of the inner ear. Sudden deafness frequently affects only one ear.

People with SSHL often discover hearing loss upon waking up in the morning. Others first notice it when they try to use the deafened ear, such as when using a phone. Still, others notice a loud, alarming "pop" just before their hearing disappears. Individuals with sudden deafness may also experience one or more of these

---

[1] "Auditory Neuropathy," National Institute on Deafness and Other Communication Disorders (NIDCD), January 26, 2018. Available online. URL: www.nidcd.nih.gov/health/auditory-neuropathy. Accessed October 9, 2024.

symptoms: a feeling of ear fullness, dizziness, and/or a ringing in their ears, such as tinnitus.

Sometimes, people with SSHL delay seeing a doctor because they think their hearing loss is due to allergies, a sinus infection, earwax plugging the ear canal, or other common conditions. However, one should consider sudden deafness symptoms a medical emergency and visit a doctor immediately. Although about half of the people with SSHL recover some or all of their hearing spontaneously, usually within one to two weeks from the onset, delaying SSHL diagnosis and treatment (when warranted) can decrease treatment effectiveness. Receiving timely treatment greatly increases the chance of recovering at least some hearing.

Experts estimate that SSHL strikes between one and six people per 5,000 every year, but the actual number of new SSHL cases each year could be much higher because SSHL often goes undiagnosed. SSHL can occur at any age but most often affects adults in their late 40s and early 50s.

WHAT CAUSES SUDDEN DEAFNESS?
A variety of disorders affecting the ear can cause SSHL, but only about 10 percent of people diagnosed with SSHL have an identifiable cause.

Some of these conditions include:
- infections
- head trauma
- autoimmune diseases
- exposure to certain drugs that treat cancer or severe infections
- blood circulation problems
- neurological disorders, such as multiple sclerosis
- disorders of the inner ear, such as Ménière disease

Most of these causes are accompanied by other medical conditions or symptoms that point to the correct diagnosis. Another factor to consider is whether hearing loss happens in one or both ears. For example, if sudden hearing loss occurs only in one ear, tumors on the auditory nerve should be ruled out as the cause. Autoimmune disease may cause SSHL in one or both ears.

HOW IS SUDDEN DEAFNESS DIAGNOSED?

If someone has sudden deafness symptoms, their doctor should rule out conductive hearing loss—hearing loss due to an obstruction in the ear, such as fluid or earwax. For sudden deafness without an obvious, identifiable cause upon examination, the doctor should perform a test called "pure tone audiometry" within a few days of the onset of symptoms to identify any sensorineural hearing loss.

With pure tone audiometry, the doctor can measure how loud different frequencies, or pitches, of sounds need to be before one can hear them. One sign of SSHL could be the loss of at least 30 decibels (decibels are a measure of sound intensity) in three connected frequencies within 72 hours. This drop would, for example, make conversational speech sound like a whisper. Patients may have more subtle, sudden changes in their hearing and may be diagnosed with other tests.

If diagnosed with sudden deafness, the doctor will probably order additional tests to try to determine an underlying cause for SSHL. These tests may include blood tests, imaging (usually magnetic resonance imaging, or MRI), and balance tests.

HOW IS SUDDEN DEAFNESS TREATED?

The most common treatment for sudden deafness, especially when the cause is unknown, is corticosteroids. Steroids can treat many disorders and usually work by reducing inflammation, decreasing swelling, and helping the body fight illness. Previously, steroids were administered in pill form. In 2011, a clinical trial supported by the National Institute on Deafness and Other Communication Disorders (NIDCD) showed that intratympanic (through the eardrum) injection of steroids was as effective as oral steroids. After this study, doctors began prescribing direct intratympanic injection of steroids into the middle ear; the medication then flows into the inner ear. The injections can be performed in the offices of many otolaryngologists and are a good option for those who cannot take oral steroids or want to avoid their side effects.

Steroids should be used as soon as possible for the best effect and may even be recommended before all test results come back.

Treatment that is delayed for more than two to four weeks is less likely to reverse or reduce permanent hearing loss.

If the doctor discovers an underlying cause of SSHL, additional treatments may be needed. For example, if SSHL is caused by an infection, the doctor may prescribe antibiotics. If one took drugs that were toxic to the ear, they may be advised to switch to another drug. If an autoimmune condition caused the immune system to attack the inner ear, the doctor may prescribe drugs that suppress the immune system.

If the hearing loss is severe, does not respond to treatment, and/or occurs in both ears, the doctor may recommend using hearing aids (to amplify sound) or even receiving cochlear implants (to directly stimulate the auditory connections in the ear that go to the brain).[1]

Section 9.7 | Hearing Problems as a Late Effect of Childhood Cancer Treatment

LATE EFFECTS OF CANCER TREATMENT

Cancer treatments may harm the body's organs, tissues, or bones and cause health problems later in life. These health problems are called "late effects."

Treatments that may cause late effects include:
- surgery
- chemotherapy
- radiation therapy
- stem cell transplant

Doctors are studying the late effects caused by cancer treatment and are working to improve cancer treatments to stop or lessen these effects. While most late effects are not life-threatening, they may cause serious problems that affect health and quality of life.

---

[1] "Sudden Deafness," National Institute on Deafness and Other Communication Disorders (NIDCD), September 14, 2018. Available online. URL: www.nidcd.nih.gov/health/sudden-deafness. Accessed October 9, 2024.

HEARING PROBLEMS AS A LATE EFFECT

Hearing problems are a late effect that is more likely to occur after treatment for certain childhood cancers. Treatment for these and other childhood cancers may cause hearing late effects:
- bone cancer
- brain tumors
- germ cell tumors
- head and neck cancers
- liver cancer
- neuroblastoma
- retinoblastoma
- soft tissue sarcoma
- cancers treated with a stem cell transplant

Radiation therapy to the brain and certain types of chemotherapy increase the risk of hearing loss. The risk of hearing loss is increased in childhood cancer survivors after treatment with the following:
- certain types of chemotherapy, such as cisplatin or high-dose carboplatin
- radiation therapy to the brain

The risk of hearing loss is greater in childhood cancer survivors who were young at the time of treatment (the younger the child, the greater the risk), were treated for a brain tumor, or received radiation therapy to the brain and chemotherapy simultaneously.

Hearing loss is the most common sign of hearing late effects. These and other signs and symptoms may be caused by hearing late effects or by other conditions:
- hearing loss
- ringing in the ears
- feeling dizzy
- excessive hardened wax in the ear

Hearing loss may occur during treatment, soon after treatment ends, or several months or years after treatment ends and may worsen over time. Talk to your child's doctor if your child experiences any of these problems.

Chronic and Acquired Disorders | 111

DIAGNOSING HEARING PROBLEMS

Certain tests and procedures are used to diagnose health problems in the ear and hearing issues. In addition to asking about your child's personal and family health history and performing a physical exam, your child's doctor may conduct the following tests and procedures:

- **Otoscopic exam.** An examination of the ear using an otoscope to inspect the ear canal and eardrum for signs of infection or hearing loss. Sometimes, the otoscope has a plastic bulb that is squeezed to release a small puff of air into the ear canal. In a healthy ear, the eardrum will move. If there is fluid behind the eardrum, it will not move.
- **Hearing test.** A hearing test can be conducted in different ways depending on the child's age. The test checks if the child can hear soft and loud sounds as well as low- and high-pitched sounds. Each ear is checked separately. The child may also be asked if they can hear the high-pitched hum of a tuning fork when it is placed behind the ear or on the forehead.

Discuss with your child's doctor whether your child needs to have tests and procedures to check for signs of hearing late effects. If tests are needed, find out how often they should be conducted.[1]

Section 9.8 | Congenital Zika Syndrome

ZIKA VIRUS INFECTION AND PREGNANCY

Zika virus infection during pregnancy can cause birth defects of the brain or eye. These birth defects can occur alone or with developmental problems in a specific pattern known as "congenital Zika

---

[1] "Late Effects of Treatment for Childhood Cancer (PDQ®)," National Cancer Institute (NCI), October 13, 2022. Available online. URL: www.cancer.gov/types/childhood-cancers/late-effects-pdq. Accessed October 9, 2024.

syndrome." The following conditions can occur in a baby with congenital Zika virus infection:
- smaller than expected head size, called "microcephaly"
- hearing loss and vision problems
- problems with brain development
- feeding problems, such as difficulty swallowing
- seizures
- decreased joint movement called "contractures"
- stiff muscles, making movement difficult

Not all babies born with congenital Zika syndrome will have all of these conditions. Some infants who do not have microcephaly at birth may develop it later. Additionally, some babies might appear healthy at birth but can develop long-term health problems as they grow.

RECOMMENDED SCREENINGS

If your baby was born with congenital Zika infection, they should receive recommended screenings even if they appear healthy. Babies and children affected by Zika virus may have lasting special needs and may require specialized care from various health-care providers and caregivers as they age.

FREQUENCY OF ZIKA-ASSOCIATED BIRTH DEFECTS

Zika virus does not cause birth defects in every baby exposed to the virus before birth (i.e., in utero). Infection with Zika virus during pregnancy simply increases the likelihood of these problems. Among people with confirmed or possible Zika infection during pregnancy in U.S. states and territories, Zika-associated birth defects occurred in about 5 percent of babies.

ZIKA SYMPTOMS AND BIRTH DEFECTS

Zika-associated birth defects can occur whether or not the pregnant person had symptoms of the infection during pregnancy. In U.S. states and territories, about 1 in 20 (5.3%) people with symptoms of Zika virus infection during pregnancy had a baby with Zika-associated birth defects, compared with about 1 in 25 (4.2%) people infected with Zika virus who had no symptoms during pregnancy.

TIMING OF ZIKA DURING PREGNANCY

Zika-associated birth defects are more common among infants born to people who were exposed early in pregnancy. The highest risk of Zika-associated birth defects is associated with infection during the first and second trimesters. In U.S. states and territories, about 2 in 25 (8%) pregnant people with confirmed Zika virus infection in the first trimester had babies with Zika-associated birth defects.

FUTURE PREGNANCIES

Zika virus infection in a person who is not pregnant does not pose a risk for future pregnancies. Similar to other infections, once a person has been infected, they are likely to be protected from future infections.[1]

---

[1] "Congenital Zika Syndrome and Other Birth Defects," Centers for Disease Control and Prevention (CDC), May 31, 2024. Available online. URL: www.cdc.gov/zika/czs/index.html. Accessed October 9, 2024.

Chapter 10 | Age-Related Hearing Loss

WHAT IS AGE-RELATED HEARING LOSS?
Age-related hearing loss (also called "presbycusis") is hearing loss that occurs gradually for many people as they grow older. It is one of the most common conditions affecting adults as they age. Approximately 15 percent of American adults (37.5 million) aged 18 and over report some trouble hearing, and about one in three people in the United States between the ages of 65 and 74 has hearing loss. Nearly half of those older than 75 have difficulty hearing.

Having trouble hearing can make it hard to understand and follow a doctor's advice, respond to warnings, and hear phones, doorbells, and smoke alarms. Hearing loss can also make it hard to enjoy talking with family and friends, leading to feelings of isolation.

Hearing loss typically occurs in both ears as we age. Because the loss is gradual, you may not realize that you have lost some of your ability to hear.

WHY DO WE LOSE OUR HEARING AS WE GET OLDER?
Many things affect our hearing as we age. For example, changes in the inner ear that can affect hearing are common. Age-related changes in the middle ear and complex changes along the nerve pathways from the ear to the brain can also affect hearing. Long-term exposure to noise and some medical conditions can also play a role. In addition, new research suggests that certain genes make some people more susceptible to hearing loss as they age.

Conditions that are more common in older people, such as high blood pressure (HBP) and diabetes, are associated with hearing loss. In addition, medications that are toxic to the sensory cells in your ears (e.g., some chemotherapy drugs) can cause hearing loss. Less commonly, abnormalities of the middle ear, such as otosclerosis, can worsen hearing with age.

CAN YOU PREVENT AGE-RELATED HEARING LOSS?

Scientists do not yet know how to prevent age-related hearing loss, but you can protect yourself from noise-induced hearing loss. Potential sources of damaging noises include loud music, headphones/earbuds used at high volume, construction equipment, fireworks, guns, lawn mowers, leaf blowers, and motorcycles. To help safeguard your hearing as you age, avoid loud noises, reduce the amount of time you are exposed to loud sounds, and protect your ears with earplugs or protective earmuffs.

HOW CAN YOU TELL IF YOU HAVE A HEARING PROBLEM?

Ask yourself the following questions. If you answer "yes" to two or more of these questions, or "sometimes" to three or more of these questions, you could have hearing loss and should consider having your hearing checked.

- Does a hearing problem cause you difficulty when listening to TV or radio?
- Does a hearing problem cause you difficulty when attending a party?
- Does a hearing problem cause you to feel frustrated when talking to members of your family?
- Does a hearing problem cause you to feel left out when you are with a group of people?
- Does a hearing problem cause you difficulty when visiting friends, relatives, or neighbors?
- Do you feel challenged by a hearing problem?
- Do you feel that any difficulty with your hearing limits or hampers your personal or social life?
- Does a hearing problem cause you to feel uncomfortable when talking to friends?
- Does a hearing problem cause you to avoid groups of people?
- Does a hearing problem cause you to visit friends, relatives, or neighbors less often than you would like?

WHAT SHOULD YOU DO IF YOU HAVE TROUBLE HEARING?

If you are concerned about your hearing, you have options for your next steps. Start by learning more about hearing loss. Depending on your symptoms, you might consider over-the-counter (OTC) hearing aids. If your symptoms are complex, or if you have questions about next steps, consider seeking advice from a hearing health-care provider. Primary care physicians, otolaryngologists, and audiologists can be important parts of your hearing health care. Each has a different type of training and expertise:

- **A primary care physician is a doctor who practices general medicine and is often our first stop for medical care.** This health-care provider can refer you to a specialist if needed and can also help determine whether you have other medical conditions that can contribute to hearing loss.
- **An otolaryngologist is a doctor who specializes in diagnosing and treating diseases of the ear, nose, throat, and neck.** An otolaryngologist, often called an "ENT," will try to find out why you are having trouble hearing and offer treatment options. Otolaryngologists often work closely with and may refer you to an audiologist.
- **An audiologist has specialized training in identifying and measuring hearing loss.** They determine where along the auditory pathway there may be a problem with hearing and recommend and provide hearing loss interventions, such as hearing aids.

WHAT TREATMENTS AND DEVICES CAN HELP?

Treatment will depend on the severity of your hearing loss, so some treatments or devices will work better for you than others. A number of devices and aids can help when you have hearing loss. Here are the most common ones:

- **Hearing aids are electronic instruments you wear in or behind your ear.** They make sounds louder. For mild to moderate hearing loss, a new category of hearing aids for adults was established in 2022 by the U.S. Food and Drug Administration (FDA). These devices may be purchased over the counter (OTC) from retail or online outlets

without seeing a health-care professional or getting a hearing test. If you have tried an OTC hearing aid without success or have trouble hearing loud sounds, consult a hearing health professional, because your hearing loss may be more severe.
- **Cochlear implants**. These are small electronic devices that are surgically implanted in the inner ear and help provide a sense of sound to people who are profoundly deaf or have severe hearing loss.
- **Assistive listening devices**. These devices include telephone and cellphone amplifiers, apps for smartphones or tablets, and closed-circuit systems (hearing loop systems) in some theaters, auditoriums, and places of worship.

HOW CAN YOUR FRIENDS AND FAMILY HELP YOU?

You and your family can work together to make living with hearing loss easier. Here are some things you can do:
- **Tell your friends and family about your hearing loss.** Explain which listening situations are hard for you.
- **Ask your friends and family to face you when they talk so that you can see their expressions and lip movements.** This may help you to understand what they are saying.
- **Ask people to speak louder, but not shout**. You may need to ask them to slow down when they speak, or to speak more clearly.
- **When you are trying to have a conversation, turn off or turn down the volume of background noise, such as the TV.**
- **Be aware of noise around you that can make hearing more difficult**. When you go to a restaurant, for example, do not sit near the kitchen or near a band playing music. Ask for seating in a quiet area. Sitting in a booth can help soften or block noise.[1]

---

[1] "Age-Related Hearing Loss (Presbycusis)," National Institute on Deafness and Other Communication Disorders (NIDCD), March 17, 2023. Available online. URL: www.nidcd.nih.gov/health/age-related-hearing-loss. Accessed October 7, 2024.

Chapter 11 | Genetic Factors in Hearing Loss

Genetic factors, including mutations in specific genes and combinations of genetic and environmental influences, play a significant role in hearing health. Early identification and intervention can help children develop communication skills and lead fulfilling lives despite hearing loss.

WHAT ARE GENES?
Genes are the basic blocks of information that all of the body's cells use to do what they are supposed to do. For example, genes tell heart cells how to beat, stomach cells how to digest food, and muscle cells how to move. Genes also contain the information for normal growth and development, and they help determine each person's physical features, such as height, eye color, and hair color.

Genes are made up of a chemical called "deoxyribonucleic acid" (DNA). DNA consists of two chemical chains joined together like rungs on a ladder. At each rung along the DNA chain, there is a part of DNA called a "base." Four different bases make up DNA, and they are A, C, T, and G, for short. The specific order, or sequence, of all the As, Cs, Ts, and Gs in DNA determines the exact information carried in each gene, similar to how a specific pattern of letters makes up the words in a sentence.

WHAT HAPPENS WHEN GENES CHANGE?
When DNA bases are missing, changed, or out of order, instructions for a gene are altered so that they cannot provide the information that cells need. These changes can cause various conditions, depending upon the types of changes and the genes involved. Some

DNA changes can cause hearing loss with other conditions (syndromic) and/or hearing loss by itself (nonsyndromic). Even among families with hearing loss in multiple relatives, DNA changes are not always found. Scientists are working to find all of the DNA-related causes of hearing loss.

HOW ARE GENES PASSED TO CHILDREN?

About half of a child's DNA comes from each parent through the egg from the mother and the sperm from the father. Thus, a child will have features similar to each parent.

Within each cell of a person's body, the genetic instructions (DNA) are packaged into larger units called "chromosomes." Each person typically has 23 pairs of chromosomes. One chromosome of each pair is from the person's mother, and the other chromosome of each pair is from the father.

WHAT ARE THE DIFFERENT WAYS GENES CAN CAUSE CONDITIONS IN CHILDREN?

Genetic conditions can be described by the chromosome that contains the gene or DNA change. If the gene is part of one of the first 22 pairs of chromosomes, called autosomes, the genetic condition is referred to as an "autosomal" condition. If the gene or DNA change is part of the X chromosome, the condition is referred to as "X-linked" or "sex-linked."

Genetic conditions can be further grouped based on who they affect in families. Changes in and around genes cause conditions to occur within members of the same family in certain patterns, called autosomal "dominant," autosomal "recessive," and X-linked "recessive."

Autosomal Dominant Conditions

"Autosomal" conditions affect both males and females equally. In "dominant" conditions, the condition is passed from parent to child. Even when only one parent has a dominant condition, the condition can still be passed on to their children. When one parent has a dominant condition, each child has a 50 percent (1 in 2) chance of having it as well. All members of the family with one gene with the dominant change will have the condition because it takes only one gene with a dominant change to cause the condition.

Autosomal Recessive Conditions

"Autosomal" conditions affect males and females equally. "Recessive" conditions are due to changes in or around genes, but they appear in families in a different way than dominant conditions. This is because people who have one recessive gene change do not have the condition. They are called "carriers." If two carriers have a child together, there is a 25 percent (1 in 4) chance that the child will inherit two recessive changed genes, one from each parent. This child will have the recessive condition. Only children who have no usual genes will have the recessive condition.

X-Linked Recessive Conditions

Hearing loss can also occur as an X-linked condition. These conditions usually affect only males. In such instances, a change in or around a gene is passed in the family through female carriers who do not have the condition. However, each son of a female carrier has a 50 percent chance of inheriting the changed gene and, therefore, of having the condition.

WHAT ARE *GJB2* AND CONNEXIN 26?

The *GJB2* gene contains the instructions for a protein called "Connexin 26." This protein is needed for a part of the ear called the "cochlea" to perform its function. The cochlea is a very complex and specialized part of the body. It needs many instructions to form and work correctly. These instructions come from many genes, including *GJB2*, *GJB3*, and *GJB6*. Changes in any one of these genes can result in hearing loss. However, unlike other autosomal recessive causes for hearing loss where severity or progression may not be predictable, *GJB2*-related hearing loss can be predicted based on the specific gene change.

Among some populations, about 50 percent of children with genetic hearing loss who do not have a syndrome will have a DNA change in the *GJB2* gene. There are many different gene changes that can cause hearing loss. Most of these changes are recessive, meaning that a person can have one usual copy of the gene and one copy of the changed *GJB2* gene and will have full hearing function. (Everyone has two *GJB2* genes, one from each parent.) However, a person who has two changed *GJB2* genes, one from each parent, will have hearing loss. This means that if both parents have just one changed *GJB2* gene, they can have a child with hearing loss, even though both parents can hear. In fact, most babies with hearing loss are born to parents who can hear.

MULTIFACTORIAL CONDITIONS

Some conditions, such as hearing loss, can be caused by a combination of genetic and non-genetic factors. These conditions are said to be "multifactorial." People who have multifactorial conditions often are born into families with no other affected members. Parents of a child with any such condition have a greater chance of having another child with the same condition than parents who do not have a child with the condition.

If a couple without hearing loss has a child with hearing loss, there are no other relatives with hearing loss, and a specific cause of the hearing loss has not been sought, the couple's chance of having another child with hearing loss is about 18 percent. However, if the child has been tested for the known genetic and non-genetic causes of hearing loss and none are identified, then the child is considered to have multifactorial hearing loss. In this case, the couple's chance of having another child with hearing loss is 3–5 percent.

MITOCHONDRIAL CONDITIONS

"Mitochondrial" conditions are different from most other genetic conditions because only the mother can pass them to her children. Also, the child receives a mixture of mitochondria that have a proportion of mitochondria with and without the changed genes. The amount of each type can be very different, ranging from all mitochondria with no gene change or all with the changed genes to a combination of everything in between. If a woman has a mitochondrial condition, the chance that she will pass it on to her children

Genetic Factors in Hearing Loss | 123

depends on the particular condition and on the amount of changed mitochondrial genes that the child receives. Fathers with a mitochondrial condition do not pass it on to their children.[1]

---

[1] "About Genetics and Hearing Loss," Centers for Disease Control and Prevention (CDC), May 15, 2024. Available online. URL: www.cdc.gov/hearing-loss-children-guide/parents-guide-genetics/about-genetics-and-hearing-loss.html. Accessed October 8, 2024.

Part 4 | Diagnosis, Prevention, and Treatment for Auditory Impairment

Chapter 12 | Diagnosis of Hearing Loss

Chapter Contents
Section 12.1—Newborn Hearing Screening...............................128
Section 12.2—Hearing Tests for Adults................................130

Section 12.1 | Newborn Hearing Screening

Do you know that a baby's hearing can be checked even before leaving the birth hospital? Many states, communities, and hospitals offer hearing screening for babies. A baby's hearing can be screened using automated auditory brainstem response (AABR), otoacoustic emissions (OAE), or both. The AABR test measures the brain's response to sound using electrodes.

Babies usually have their hearing screened while still in the hospital, either in the nursery or in their mother's room.

IMPORTANCE OF EARLY HEARING SCREENING

Hearing screening is easy and not painful. In fact, babies are often asleep while being screened. It takes a very short time—usually only a few minutes. Sometimes the screening is repeated while the babies are still in the hospital or shortly after they leave the hospital.

FOLLOW-UP TESTING FOR BABIES WHO DO NOT PASS SCREENING

Babies who do not pass hearing screening should be tested by an audiologist. An audiologist is a person trained to test hearing. This person will conduct additional testing to determine whether there is a hearing loss. An audiologist can perform many kinds of tests to determine if a baby has hearing loss, how much hearing loss there is, and what type it is.

EARLY INTERVENTION FOR BABIES WITH HEARING LOSS

Finding a hearing loss early and getting into a program that helps babies with hearing loss (beginning before a baby is 6 months old) helps a child to achieve the following:
- Communicate better with others.
- Do well in school.
- Get along with other children.

Intervention services are types of programs and resources available for children and their families. An intervention might be:
- meeting with a professional (or team) who is trained to work with children who have a hearing loss and their families

- working with a professional (or team) who can help a family and child learn to communicate
- fitting a baby with a hearing device, such as a hearing aid
- joining family support groups
- accessing other resources available to children with hearing loss and their families

RESCREENING PROCESS FOR BABIES

All babies who do not pass their first hearing screening should be rescreened one to two weeks later or have a complete hearing test. The baby's doctor or the hospital where the baby was born can provide information on where to take the child for the hearing rescreen or test.

COMPREHENSIVE HEARING TESTING BY AUDIOLOGISTS

An expert (audiologist) trained to test the baby's hearing will perform a complete hearing test (audiology evaluation). An audiologist who works with children is sometimes called a "pediatric audiologist."

An audiology evaluation is more than just one test. The audiologist might use tests such as:
- assessing the function of the baby's outer and middle ear
- measuring the baby's reactions to sounds
- evaluating how the ears respond to sound
- testing the ear nerve's response to sound

The audiologist will ask questions about the baby's birth history, ear infections, hearing loss in the family, and perceptions of how well the baby hears.

The results from all the tests, along with the information provided, will be examined collectively, and the audiologist will make a diagnosis. With permission, the audiologist will share the results with the baby's doctor and possibly an ear, nose, and throat doctor (referred to as an "otolaryngologist"). These professionals will collaborate to enhance understanding of the baby's condition. They might recommend further evaluations by other specialists, such as an eye doctor (ophthalmologist), a geneticist, or others.[1]

---

[1] "Newborn Hearing Screening," Centers for Disease Control and Prevention (CDC), May 15, 2024. Available online. URL: www.cdc.gov/hearing-loss-children-guide/parents-guide/newborn-hearing-screening.html. Accessed October 9, 2024.

Section 12.2 | Hearing Tests for Adults

Hearing loss in older adults is common. About one-third of adults over the age of 65 have some hearing loss, usually the sensorineural type. If you are diagnosed with hearing loss, there are steps you can take that may help treat or manage the condition.

Other names include:
- audiometry
- audiography
- audiogram
- sound test
- audiologic tests

WHAT ARE HEARING TESTS?

Hearing tests measure how well you are able to hear. They can help diagnose hearing loss, determine its severity, and identify which part of your hearing is not functioning properly.

Hearing depends on a series of steps that change sound waves into electrical signals that your brain understands as sounds. Hearing loss occurs when there is a problem with any of these steps:

1. Sound waves enter your outer ear and travel to your eardrum in your middle ear.
2. The sound waves vibrate your eardrum, which sends the vibrations to tiny bones that amplify the vibrations.
3. The vibrating bones create tiny waves in the fluid inside your cochlea. The cochlea is a snail-shaped structure in your inner ear, lined with sensory cells that have hair-like structures. When the hair cells move with the fluid waves, they create electrical signals.
4. Your auditory (hearing) nerve carries the electrical signals from your inner ear to your brain, which converts them into sounds you can recognize and understand.

There are three main types of hearing loss:
- **Conductive hearing loss**. It happens when sound waves cannot reach your inner ear. Earwax or abnormal fluid in your ear may be blocking the path, or a hole in your

eardrum may prevent it from vibrating. Medical treatment or surgery can often improve hearing.
- **Sensorineural hearing loss (also called "nerve deafness")**. It occurs when there is damage to the inner ear or the auditory nerve. This type of hearing loss ranges from mild (difficulty hearing certain sounds) to profound (not hearing any sound). The loss is usually permanent, but it can improve with hearing aids or other devices.
- **Mixed hearing loss**. It is a combination of both sensorineural and conductive hearing loss.

WHAT ARE THEY USED FOR?
Hearing tests are used to check for hearing loss and determine its severity and type.

WHY DO I NEED A HEARING TEST?
You may need a hearing test if you have signs of hearing loss, such as:
- having trouble hearing over the phone
- having difficulty understanding what other people are saying, especially in a noisy environment
- needing to turn up the TV volume so loud that others complain
- thinking that others always seem to mumble
- having trouble hearing high-pitched sounds and voices
- hearing a ringing or other unusual sound in your ears (tinnitus)

If your workplace is noisy, you may need to have your hearing checked every year.

If you use a hearing aid or have had surgery for your hearing, you may need a hearing test to see whether your hearing has improved.

WHAT HAPPENS DURING A HEARING TEST?
Your primary care provider may use a general screening test to check your hearing. This is usually a whisper test to see how well you can hear whispered words in each ear.

If the test shows you may have a hearing problem or if you notice you have trouble hearing, your provider may conduct additional hearing tests or refer you to a hearing specialist, such as:
- **An audiologist**. A health-care professional trained to test your hearing, diagnose hearing loss, and provide hearing devices and services to improve hearing.
- **An otolaryngologist (ENT)**. A doctor who specializes in treating diseases of the ears, nose, throat, and head and neck.
- **Hearing aid specialists, who can perform basic hearing tests and fit you for hearing aids**. If you have a hearing aid, tests can check whether it is helping you sufficiently. If you are unsure where to have your hearing tested, talk with your primary care provider.

TYPES OF HEARING TESTS

There are several types of hearing tests. These are some of the more common types:

Audiometry Tests

Audiometry tests check your ability to hear tones or words at different pitches and volumes. For these tests, you will wear headphones and sit in a soundproof room. The tests may include:
- **A pure-tone test**. This is the most common screening test for hearing loss. It tests for the quietest sounds you can hear at different pitches. During the test, the following will occur:
  - Your headphones will play a series of high and low tones, some of which will be loud and some very soft.
  - Each time you hear a tone, you will raise your hand, push a button, or say that you hear the sound.
- **Speech test or speech discrimination test**. This test checks how well you can hear people talking. It can show how much a hearing aid might help you. During the test, the following will occur:
  - You will hear simple words at different levels of loudness, and some words will be spoken over noise.
  - You will repeat the words that you hear.

- **Tuning fork tests or bone conduction tests.** These tests can help distinguish between nerve problems in your inner ear (sensorineural hearing loss) and fluid or wax that makes it hard to hear (conductive hearing loss). They can also show if one ear hears better than the other. A tuning fork is a two-pronged metal device. When it is tapped, it vibrates and produces a sound. Tuning forks are mostly used by primary care providers. Audiologists and otolaryngologists may use special devices for bone conduction testing. The general steps are the same:
  - The provider will place the tuning fork or device behind your ear or on your head.
  - The tuning fork or device will vibrate, causing your skull bones to vibrate gently.
  - The vibrations travel through your bones directly into your inner ear, bypassing the outer and middle ear.

Tympanometry Test

A tympanometry test checks how your eardrum and the bones in your middle ear are functioning:
- A small device will be placed in your ear.
- The device will send air and sound into your ear, causing your eardrum to move. You will feel the air pressure inside your ear.
- A machine records the movements of your eardrum on graphs called "tympanograms."

If your eardrum does not move normally, you may have fluid or wax buildup in your ear, a hole in your eardrum, a tumor in your ear, middle ear bones that do not vibrate well, or another problem in your middle ear.

Otoacoustic Emissions Test

An otoacoustic emissions (OAE) test checks for damage in the hair cells in your cochlea:
- **A small device will be placed in your ear.** It can produce sound and measure sound.

- **Sound from the device causes the fluid in your cochlea to ripple, moving the hair cells.** When the hair cells move, they create vibrations that generate their own sound.
- **The device measures OAE to determine the health of hair cells.** If the test shows little or no OAEs, you have sensorineural hearing loss.

WHAT DO THE RESULTS MEAN?

The results of hearing tests show if your hearing is normal or if you have hearing loss. You will usually receive your results right after your tests are completed.

If you have hearing loss, the results will show how severe it is, which ear is affected more, and whether you have conductive, sensorineural, or both types of hearing loss:

- **With conductive hearing loss, your provider may be able to treat the cause and restore your hearing.** Your treatment will depend on what is blocking sound from reaching your inner ear. It may include removing wax, draining fluid, or surgery to fix problems with your eardrum or ear bones.
- **With sensorineural hearing loss, your hearing loss cannot be treated, but you may be able to use hearing aids or have surgery to implant a device to improve your hearing.** If your hearing cannot be improved, assistive devices are available to help with daily living. For example, there are devices to help you use the phone and to alert you to doorbells, alarms, and other sounds.

In certain cases, more tests may be needed to diagnose the cause of the hearing loss. If you have questions about your test results, talk with your health-care provider.[1]

---

[1] MedlinePlus, "Hearing Tests for Adults," National Institutes of Health (NIH), October 25, 2023. Available online. URL: https://medlineplus.gov/lab-tests/hearing-tests-for-adults. Accessed October 7, 2024.

Chapter 13 | Preventing Noise-Induced Auditory Loss

Chapter Contents
Section 13.1—Protecting Your Hearing from Noise-Induced Damage........136
Section 13.2—Selecting and Using Effective Hearing Protectors 138
Section 13.3—Strategies for Preventing Noise-Induced Hearing Loss in Students 140
Section 13.4—Strategies for Teaching Children to Protect Their Hearing....143

Section 13.1 | Protecting Your Hearing from Noise-Induced Damage

HEARING LOSS
Hearing loss can occur:
- in children and affect communication, language, and social skills
- in occupational settings and result in permanent injury for workers
- due to loud noise near the ear or repeated exposure to loud noise

Exposure to loud noise can lead to noise-induced hearing loss. This can be caused by participating in activities that produce harmful sound levels or by repeated exposure to loud sounds.

Some examples of noisy activities include:
- watching summer fireworks on the 4th of July
- mowing the lawn
- using power tools
- watching a sports game and cheering on your favorite team
- attending a concert

Recognize early signs of noise-induced hearing loss and take steps to protect your hearing.

PREVALENCE
An estimated 12.5 percent of children and adolescents aged 6–19 years (approximately 5.2 million) and 17 percent of adults aged 20–69 years (approximately 26 million) have suffered permanent damage to their hearing from excessive exposure to noise.

CAUSES
Hearing loss can result from damage to structures and/or nerve fibers in the inner ear that respond to sound. Noise-induced hearing loss is usually caused by exposure to excessively loud sounds and cannot be medically or surgically corrected. It can result from

one-time exposure to a very loud sound, blast, or impulse or from listening to loud sounds over an extended period.

PREVENTION

Hearing loss caused by exposure to loud sound is preventable. To reduce the risk of noise-induced hearing loss, adults and children can do the following:

- Understand that noise-induced hearing loss can lead to communication difficulties, learning difficulties, pain or ringing in the ears (tinnitus), distorted or muffled hearing, and an inability to hear some environmental sounds and warning signals.
- Identify sources of loud sounds (such as gas-powered lawnmowers, snowmobiles, power tools, gunfire, or music) that can contribute to hearing loss and try to reduce exposure.
- Adopt behaviors to protect hearing:
  - Avoid or limit exposure to excessively loud sounds.
  - Turn down the volume of the music system.
  - Move away from the source of loud sounds when possible.
  - Use hearing protection devices when it is not feasible to avoid exposure to loud sounds or reduce them to a safe level.
  - Seek hearing evaluation by a licensed audiologist or other qualified professional, especially if there is concern about potential hearing loss.[1]

---

[1] "Preventing Noise-Induced Hearing Loss," Centers for Disease Control and Prevention (CDC), May 15, 2024. Available online. URL: www.cdc.gov/hearing-loss-children/about/preventing-noise-induced-hearing-loss.html. Accessed October 10, 2024.

Section 13.2 | Selecting and Using Effective Hearing Protectors

UNDERSTANDING HEARING PROTECTION
Effective hearing protection is crucial for safeguarding workers from noise-induced hearing loss. Employers should not rely on personal protective equipment (PPE) alone to control hazards when other effective control options are available. Employers should implement engineering and administrative controls first to reduce worker noise exposure. PPE is generally less effective than elimination, substitution, and engineering controls. Hearing protection is often:
- inadequately chosen
- worn incorrectly
- used inconsistently

Employers can avoid these pitfalls by selecting appropriate hearing protectors and providing proper training. Training should ensure workers know where to use hearing protection and how to use it correctly. Follow hearing protection best practices:
- **Offer varied hearing protection options.** Provide workers with a variety of hearing protection options that will reduce noise exposure to less than the recommended exposure limit (REL) of 85 decibels A-weighted (dBA), a unit that reflects the ear's sensitivity to different frequencies of sound.
- **Select hearing protectors that are comfortable and compatible with the job.** Reevaluate hearing protector options when working conditions and noise exposures change or when a worker develops a hearing shift.
- **Train management as well as workers.** Identify unique motivations for each group to prioritize hearing safety.

CHOOSING HEARING PROTECTORS
Hearing protection comes in many styles, materials, colors, and sizes. The main types of hearing protectors include the following:
- **Earplugs.** Devices that slide snugly into the ear canal. They can be formable (such as foam, which expands to

fit the contour of the canal), preformed (which is already shaped to fit most ears), or custom (which uses an impression of the worker's ear to make a device uniquely fitted to that person).
- **Earmuffs.** Devices that completely surround the outer ear and are held in place by a headband or attached to a hard hat.
- **Canal caps.** Devices that cover the entrance to the ear canals and are held in place by a lightweight band.

Some hearing protectors have special features that are helpful for certain types of noise or work situations. Examples of these features in hearing protectors include the following:
- **Flat attenuation.** These hearing protectors (sometimes called "musicians' earplugs") reduce noise equally across all frequency bands, preserving the fidelity of the sound.
- **Nonlinear.** These hearing protectors (which include level-dependent and sound restoration hearing protectors) allow quiet sounds to pass through but block loud sounds.
- **Communication technologies.** These hearing protectors have built-in microphones and speakers, making it easier to talk to other workers in a noisy environment.

KNOW HOW MUCH HEARING PROTECTION YOU WILL NEED

The most basic consideration is the noise exposure level. However, most workers need 10 dB or less sound reduction to bring their exposure down to a safe level. Almost any hearing protector, when fit correctly, can reduce noise by 10 dB. Keep the following guidelines in mind:
- Aim for just enough noise reduction to bring exposure down to 75–85 dBA.
- Avoid overprotection—too much sound reduction can make workers less aware of their surroundings.
- Workers might take off their hearing protectors to hear properly.

- Provide double hearing protection (earmuffs over earplugs) for workers exposed to noise levels of 100 dBA or greater or impulse sounds.
- Fit test workers to ensure their hearing protectors are providing the right level of noise reduction.

TIPS FOR TRAINING WORKERS ABOUT HEARING PROTECTION
- If workers need to wear hearing protectors, they should know where to put them and how to use them correctly.
- Train management as well as workers.
- Identify unique motivations for each group to prioritize hearing safety.
- Regularly reevaluate and implement additional training if needed.[1]

Section 13.3 | Strategies for Preventing Noise-Induced Hearing Loss in Students

Schools can take several steps to prevent noise-induced hearing loss, including limiting exposure to excessive noise on school property, screening for existing noise-induced hearing loss, and teaching students how to protect their hearing.

ESTABLISH POLICIES THAT PROMOTE THE HEARING HEALTH OF STUDENTS AND STAFF
School districts can adopt policies and procedures to minimize excessive noise during the school day and protect the hearing of their students and staff. For example, schools can take the following actions:
- Eliminate or reduce construction and maintenance activities during school hours.
- Set noise level standards for events such as school dances.

---

[1] National Institute for Occupational Safety and Health (NIOSH), "Provide Hearing Protection," Centers for Disease Control and Prevention (CDC), February 16, 2024. Available online. URL: www.cdc.gov/niosh/noise/prevent/ppe.html. Accessed October 9, 2024.

- Ensure that hearing protection devices are available to students, instruct them on their proper use, and require these devices in classes or activities where students are exposed to potentially unsafe noise levels (e.g., music classes, marching band, industrial arts, and technology education classes).
- Implement policies consistent with National Institute for Occupational Safety and Health (NIOSH) recommendations (www.cdc.gov/niosh/docs/98-126) to support hearing loss prevention programs for school employees.

ESTABLISH AND MAINTAIN ROUTINE HEARING SCREENING FOR ALL STUDENTS

Many schools provide hearing screening as part of required student health assessments. Hearing screening, especially at an early age, provides the opportunity to detect a student's hearing loss or previously unrecognized hearing loss and intervene to limit further loss and improve learning. According to the American Academy of Pediatrics (AAP), hearing screening should be conducted:

- at school entry for all children
- at least once at ages 6, 8, and 10
- at least once during middle school
- at least once during high school
- for any student entering a new school system without evidence of a previous hearing screening

Hearing screening might be required more often for students with other known health or learning needs, speech, language, or developmental delays, or a family history of early hearing loss.

Hearing screening programs should be consistent with the AAP Criteria for Successful Screening Programs in Schools to ensure that all necessary standards and practices are met for effective screening and support for students with hearing loss.

- Screening tests are accurate and reliable.
- The school hearing screening site is suitable and appropriate for screening.
- People who screen students' hearing are well-trained and qualified professionals.

- Community and health-care provider referral mechanisms are in place so that those with identified hearing loss can receive additional evaluation, diagnosis, and appropriate treatment if needed.
- Student screening results are communicated effectively by the school to students, parents, and health-care providers.
- Effective treatment and early intervention benefit those with identified hearing loss or hearing difficulties.
- Appropriate educational interventions are implemented to reduce the negative effects of hearing loss on student learning.
- The benefits of hearing screening outweigh the cost of implementing the screening program.

Screening programs might not capture all cases of noise-induced hearing loss. Any student or school personnel reporting hearing difficulties or tinnitus (especially after loud sound exposure) should be referred to an audiologist for further evaluation.

IMPLEMENT HEARING LOSS PREVENTION EDUCATION

Education about noise and its effects on hearing, health, and learning can begin in elementary school. Studies have shown that people who are educated about noise-induced hearing loss and hearing loss prevention are more likely to use hearing protection devices in future occupational and recreational settings. Comprehensive hearing loss prevention programs include instruction for students on:
- normal hearing (auditory) function
- types of hearing loss and their causes
- common sources of noise that can contribute to hearing loss
- noise and its effects on hearing and quality of life
- warning signs of noise-induced hearing loss
- recommendations for preventing hearing loss

Hearing loss prevention education can be part of a school's health education curriculum or integrated across curricula and

other school programs by health professionals and trained volunteers, teachers, and parents. Below are a few examples of how to enhance hearing loss prevention and education:
- School nurses, physicians, audiologists, speech-language pathologists (SLPs), or well-trained volunteers can help provide accurate information and interactive activities.
- Teachers can be taught how to reduce loud sounds in the school environment and model good hearing protection behavior and attitudes.
- Education can also be provided for parents, encouraging them to practice hearing loss prevention at home and to teach it to their children.[1]

Section 13.4 | Strategies for Teaching Children to Protect Their Hearing

Whether you are a teacher, community leader, or health professional, your regular interactions with kids provide you with unique opportunities to help shape their healthy hearing habits for life. Just as wearing sunscreen can protect against sun damage, these healthy hearing habits can protect kids from hearing loss caused by loud noises. When talking to kids about noise and hearing loss, remind them to take the following actions:
- Lower the volume.
- Move away from the noise.
- Wear hearing protectors, such as earplugs or earmuffs.

Here are some ideas for teaching kids about noise-induced hearing loss and how to protect their hearing.

---

[1] "Promoting Hearing Health in Schools," Centers for Disease Control and Prevention (CDC), August 26, 2015. Available online. URL: www.cdc.gov/healthyschools/noise/promoting.htm. Accessed October 11, 2024.

SCHOOLS
Science and Health Teachers
- If your school has a decibel meter, ask students to measure noise levels in various parts of the school, such as the cafeteria, music room, hallways, and gym.
- Suggest science fair projects that explore how loud sounds can damage hearing.
- Review the anatomy of the ear and educate students about safe sound levels and those that can cause noise-induced hearing loss.
- Teach by example: show your students how you protect your hearing by using hearing protectors.

Music Teachers
- Integrate noise-induced hearing loss prevention messages into band and orchestra classes and rehearsals.
- Show students how to use hearing protection, specifically hearing protection for musicians.
- When possible, turn down amplifiers and other sound equipment.
- Make sure speakers and amplifiers are not positioned near students during performances.

School Nurses
- Include information about healthy hearing habits in email newsletters or other information sent to teachers and parents.

School Administrators
- Consider purchasing a decibel meter to measure the noise levels of gym classes, sporting events, the cafeteria, music classes, and hallways between classes. Make students aware of how noisy these areas are and point out the potential risk to their hearing. Work with students and teachers to reduce the noise level of the loudest areas.
- Share hearing protection devices in classrooms that regularly have potentially unsafe noise levels—such as music classes and industrial arts.

- Discourage "noise competitions" at sporting or other events.
- Explore opportunities to partner with local drugstores or sporting goods stores to distribute earplugs at school concerts, sporting events, and noisy social events.
- Encourage science and music teachers to include classroom activities on noise-induced hearing loss.
- Get the community involved in helping to reduce noise. Write an article for your school newsletter or listserv (email distribution list).

AFTER-SCHOOL AND YOUTH PROGRAMS, COMMUNITY CENTER STAFF, AND OTHER EDUCATORS

- Schedule a session on noise and hearing loss with your youth program.
- Teach kids about noise levels.
- Ensure that sound levels are safe during events such as dances and talent shows.
- Train your staff to implement safe hearing practices.

PEDIATRICIAN OFFICES, CLINICS, AND OTHER HEALTHCARE FACILITIES

- Discuss with parents and preteens the conditions that affect hearing health.
- During annual exams:
  - Ask your young patients how loud and how frequently they listen to music through headphones or earbuds.
  - Explain the dangers of noise-induced hearing loss.
  - Be specific about the sources of harmful noise.
  - Urge parents and preteens to obtain hearing protectors so they can continue to enjoy the sounds they love while protecting their hearing.
- Inform parents about hearing screenings and alert them to potential problems if their child complains about hearing issues or if they have been exposed to loud noises.

By fostering awareness and implementing practical strategies, educators and health professionals can significantly contribute to protecting children from noise-induced hearing loss.[1]

---

[1] "Tips for Teaching Kids about Noise-Induced Hearing Loss," National Institute on Deafness and Other Communication Disorders (NIDCD), April 22, 2019. Available online. URL: www.noisyplanet.nidcd.nih.gov/educators/tips-to-teach-kids. Accessed October 9, 2024.

Chapter 14 | Intervention and Treatment for Auditory Impairment

Chapter Contents
Section 14.1—Intervention Strategies for Children with Hearing Loss.......148
Section 14.2—Medications and Surgery for Hearing Loss in Children 152
Section 14.3—Steroid Treatments for Sudden Deafness 153
Section 14.4—Gene Therapy for Hearing Loss...........................155

Section 14.1 | Intervention Strategies for Children with Hearing Loss

TREATMENT AND INTERVENTION OVERVIEW
No single treatment or intervention for hearing loss is the answer for every child or family. Intervention plans will include close monitoring, follow-ups, and any changes needed along the way. There are many options for children with hearing loss and their families.

Treatment and intervention options for hearing loss in children include:
- working with a professional (or team) who can help a child and family learn to communicate
- getting a hearing device, such as a hearing aid
- joining support groups
- taking advantage of other resources available to children with hearing loss and their families

TREATMENT AND INTERVENTION TYPES
Intervention Services
Early Intervention (0–3 years)
Hearing loss can affect a child's ability to develop speech, language, and social skills. The earlier a child who is deaf or hard of hearing starts receiving services, the more likely the child's communication (speech or sign language) and social skills will reach their full potential.

Early intervention program services help young children with hearing loss learn communication and other important skills. Research shows that early intervention services can greatly improve a child's development.

Babies who are diagnosed with hearing loss should begin to receive intervention services as soon as possible, but no later than six months of age.

There are many services available through the Individuals with Disabilities Education Improvement Act of 2004 (IDEA 2004). Services for children from birth through 36 months of age are called "Early Intervention" or "Part C services." Even if your child has not been diagnosed with hearing loss, they may be eligible for early

Intervention and Treatment for Auditory Impairment

intervention treatment services. The IDEA 2004 states that children under the age of three years (36 months) who are at risk of having developmental delays may be eligible for services. These services are provided through an early intervention system in your state. Through this system, you can request an evaluation.

Special Education (3–22 years)
Special education is instruction specifically designed to address the educational and related developmental needs of older children with disabilities or those experiencing developmental delays. Services for these children are provided through the public school system and are available through the Individuals with Disabilities Education Improvement Act of 2004 (IDEA 2004), Part B.

Assistive Technology
Many people who are deaf or hard of hearing have some hearing. The amount of hearing a deaf or hard of hearing person has is called "residual hearing." Technology does not "cure" hearing loss but may help a child with hearing loss to make the most of their residual hearing. For those parents who choose to have their child use technology, there are many options, including:
- hearing aids
- cochlear or brainstem implants
- bone-anchored hearing aids
- other assistive devices

Hearing Aids
Hearing aids make sounds louder. They can be worn by people of any age, including infants. Babies with hearing loss may understand sounds better using hearing aids. This may give them the chance to learn speech skills at a young age.

There are many styles of hearing aids, and they can help many types of hearing loss. Behind-the-ear hearing aids are usually better suited to young children because they are better suited to growing ears.

Cochlear and Auditory Brainstem Implants
A cochlear implant may help many children with severe to profound hearing loss—even very young children. It provides that child with

a way to hear when a hearing aid is not sufficient. Unlike a hearing aid, cochlear implants do not make sounds louder. Instead, they send sound signals directly to the hearing nerve.

Individuals with severe to profound hearing loss due to an absent or very small hearing nerve or severely abnormal inner ear (cochlea) may not benefit from a hearing aid or cochlear implant. Instead, an auditory brainstem implant may provide some hearing. An auditory brainstem implant directly stimulates the hearing pathways in the brainstem, bypassing the inner ear and hearing nerve.

Both cochlear and brainstem implants have two main parts: the parts that are placed inside the inner ear, the cochlea, or base of the brain, the brainstem during surgery; and the parts outside the ear that send sounds to the parts inside the ear.

Bone-Anchored Hearing Aids

This type of hearing aid can be considered when a child has conductive, mixed, or unilateral hearing loss and is specifically suitable for children who cannot otherwise wear "in-the-ear" or "behind-the-ear" hearing aids.

Other Assistive Devices

Besides hearing aids, there are other devices that help people with hearing loss. Examples of other assistive devices include the following:

- **Frequency modulation (FM) systems**. An FM system is a device that helps people with hearing loss hear in background noise. FM is the same type of signal used for radios. These systems send sound from a microphone used by someone speaking to a person wearing the receiver. FM is sometimes used with hearing aids. An extra piece is attached to the hearing aid that works with the FM system.
- **Captioning**. Many television programs, videos, and DVDs are captioned. Television sets made after 1993 are designed to show captioning. You do not have to buy anything special. Captions show the conversation spoken in the soundtrack of a program on the bottom of the television screen.

Intervention and Treatment for Auditory Impairment | 151

Other devices include:
- text messaging
- telephone amplifiers
- flashing and vibrating alarms
- audio loop systems
- infrared listening devices
- portable sound amplifiers
- TTY (text telephone or teletypewriter)

LEARNING LANGUAGE

Without extra help, children with hearing loss have difficulty learning language, which can put them at risk for other delays. Families who have children with hearing loss often need to change their communication habits or learn special skills (such as sign language) to help their children learn language. These skills can be used together with hearing aids, cochlear or auditory brainstem implants, and other devices that help children hear.

FAMILY SUPPORT SERVICES

For many parents, their child's hearing loss is unexpected. Parents sometimes need time and support to adapt to the child's hearing loss.

Parents of children with recently identified hearing loss can seek different kinds of support. Support encompasses anything that assists a family and may include advice, information, opportunities to connect with other parents of children with hearing loss, access to a mentor who is fluent in sign language, help in finding childcare or transportation, giving parents time for personal relaxation, or simply offering a supportive listener.[1]

---

[1] "Treatment and Intervention for Hearing Loss," Centers for Disease Control and Prevention (CDC), May 15, 2024. Available online. URL: www.cdc.gov/hearing-loss-children/treatment. Accessed October 9, 2024.

Section 14.2 | Medications and Surgery for Hearing Loss in Children

Medications or surgery may also help make the most of a child's hearing. This is especially true for outer or conductive hearing loss, which involves a part of the outer or middle ear that is not functioning in the usual way.

CONDUCTIVE HEARING LOSS AND EAR INFECTIONS
One type of conductive hearing loss can be caused by a chronic ear infection. A chronic ear infection is a buildup of fluid behind the eardrum in the middle ear space. Ear infections are common among all children, including those who have hearing loss. Even young infants can experience them. If you think your child has an ear infection, it is important to take them to your child's doctor. For a child with hearing loss, an ear infection can further decrease their hearing. Please discuss this with your child's doctor and your care team.

Most ear infections can be treated with medication or careful observation. If your child's doctor identifies an ear infection, they may prescribe one or more medications for your child to take. Infections that do not resolve with medication can be treated with a simple surgery that involves placing a tiny tube into the child's eardrum to drain the fluid.

STRUCTURAL ISSUES AND SURGERY
Another type of conductive hearing loss is caused by a part of the outer or middle ear that did not form correctly while the child was developing in the mother's womb. Several parts of the outer and middle ear need to work together to transmit sound to the inner ear. If any of these parts did not form correctly, there may be hearing loss in that ear. This can be improved and perhaps even corrected with surgery performed by an ear, nose, and throat doctor (otolaryngologist).

COCHLEAR IMPLANTS FOR SEVERE HEARING LOSS
A cochlear implant can help a person with severe to profound hearing loss. It provides a way for a person to hear when a hearing aid is

insufficient. Unlike a hearing aid, cochlear implants do not amplify sounds. Instead, they send sound signals directly to the hearing nerve. These signals bypass parts of the inner ear (hair cells) that are not functioning correctly. A cochlear implant does not "cure" hearing loss but allows a person with hearing loss to discern sounds.

THE COCHLEAR IMPLANT PROCEDURE

Surgery is necessary to implant a cochlear device. The procedure takes a few hours, and general anesthesia is required. Typically, children and adults receiving a cochlear implant need to stay in the hospital for one night following the surgery. It takes about 3–5 weeks for the skin over the surgery site to heal, but children usually return to normal activities in about 10 days.

If your child receives a cochlear implant, they will need to return to the audiologist four to six weeks after surgery to have the device activated. After the cochlear implant is turned on, your child may require several additional visits to ensure the implant is correctly adjusted.

SUPPORT FROM SPEECH-LANGUAGE PATHOLOGISTS

Your doctors and audiologist may also recommend that your child undergo training with a speech-language pathologist (SLP). A SLP is a professional trained in how children learn language and can teach children to use speech and language effectively. This training will help your child understand the new sounds they hear with a cochlear implant.[1]

Section 14.3 | Steroid Treatments for Sudden Deafness

SUDDEN DEAFNESS

Injecting steroids into the middle ear works just as well as taking them orally to restore hearing for patients with sudden deafness.

---

[1] "Intervention Options," Centers for Disease Control and Prevention (CDC), May 15, 2024. Available online. URL: www.cdc.gov/hearing-loss-children-guide/parents-guide/intervention-options.html. Accessed October 10, 2024.

This finding, the result of a large clinical trial comparing the therapies, will help doctors choose the best treatment for patients with this condition.

Sudden deafness, also called "sudden sensorineural hearing loss," is an emergency medical condition that affects several thousand people annually, usually between the ages of 40 and 60. It often arises without an obvious cause and occurs in one ear all at once or over a period of up to three days. Oral steroids, such as prednisone, are typically prescribed over the course of two weeks to restore hearing. There is only a two- to four-week window of time for treatment before hearing loss becomes permanent.

INTRATYMPANIC STEROID TREATMENT

Doctors have begun injecting steroids directly into the middle ear, a procedure known as "intratympanic treatment." This technique is thought to deliver more of the drug to the ear and to avoid some of the side effects that can accompany oral steroids. The side effects of oral therapy can be mild, such as weight gain, mood changes, and sleep disruption, or more serious, such as high blood pressure (HBP) and elevated blood sugar. Side effects of injected steroids are usually local, such as ear infection and vertigo.

To investigate, Dr. Steven Rauch of Harvard Medical School and the Massachusetts Eye and Ear Infirmary led a team of investigators from 16 medical centers nationwide in a clinical trial involving more than 250 patients. The trial was funded by the National Institutes of Health's (NIH) National Institute on Deafness and Other Communication Disorders (NIDCD). The results were published in the May 25, 2011, issue of the *Journal of the American Medical Association*.

The study tested the treatments as they are usually administered in the clinic. For oral steroid therapy, patients received 60 milligrams of prednisone for 14 days, followed by a tapering-off period of five days. The other group was given 40 milligrams of methylprednisolone injected directly through the eardrum four times over the course of two weeks. The study followed the recovery of these patients for six months, measuring the success of the treatments based on hearing tests at the first and second weeks, and at months two and six.

Under both regimens, patients recovered their hearing to about the same extent at two and six months. The oral steroid patients experienced typical symptoms, such as changes in sleep, mood, and appetite. The injected steroid patients had pain at the injection site and vertigo; a few experienced ear infections and a perforated eardrum. Most symptoms cleared up by six months. Nevertheless, the findings indicated that while the treatments were equally effective, they might not be equally appropriate for every patient.

"The comfort, cost, and convenience of oral steroid treatment are preferable to intratympanic treatment," says Dr. Rauch, "but injected steroids are an equally effective alternative for people who, for medical reasons, cannot take the oral steroids. People with sudden deafness should discuss the risks and benefits of both treatments with their doctor."[1]

Section 14.4 | Gene Therapy for Hearing Loss

Hearing loss is one of the most common communication disorders in the world. Aging, exposure to loud noise, head trauma, genetic mutations, some medications, and bacterial infections can all lead to hearing loss.

"As patients lose their hearing, they become more socially withdrawn because they do not want to embarrass themselves in front of their family members and friends. There is a significant impact on the patient's health as well as overall quality of life," said Dr. Wade Chien, an otolaryngology surgeon-scientist in the National Institute on Deafness and Other Communication Disorders' (NIDCD) Inner Ear Gene Therapy Program.

When a sound wave enters the ear, it travels through a narrow passage called the "ear canal." There, it meets the eardrum. The

---

[1] News and Events, "Steroid Treatments Equally Effective against Sudden Deafness," National Institutes of Health (NIH), June 6, 2011. Available online. URL: www.nih.gov/news-events/nih-research-matters/steroid-treatments-equally-effective-against-sudden-deafness. Accessed October 10, 2024.

sound waves strike the eardrum, which causes three tiny bones in the middle ear to vibrate. The vibrations travel to the cochlea, a fluid-filled structure shaped like a snail's spiral shell, which activates the sensory cells in the inner ear called "hair cells."

Hair cells translate the vibrations into electrical signals, which auditory nerve fibers send to the brain. The hair cells can detect a wide range of frequencies. Additionally, the vestibular organs in the inner ear help maintain a person's balance.

Hearing aids are one treatment option for patients with mild to moderate hearing loss. However, only 14 percent of the U.S. population with hearing loss wears hearing aids. Dr. Chien thinks people are not aware of the problems that hearing loss causes, so they do not appreciate the health benefits of hearing.

"Fortunately, this is rapidly changing" due to research, he said. "It's my hope more and more people will realize the importance of treatment for hearing loss."

Some people, particularly those with severe hearing loss, do not find hearing aids effective. Many of Dr. Chien's patients with severe hearing loss say hearing aids make sounds louder, not clearer.

Dr. Chien said cochlear implants are another treatment option for these patients. A cochlear implant is a device that stimulates the auditory nerve. The implant has external and internal parts. The external part includes a microphone, which relays information to the internal part, which transmits it to the cochlea.

"While hearing aids and cochlear implants are useful therapeutic options for patients with hearing loss, they are not perfect," Dr. Chien said.

The lack of effective treatments inspired him to find new ones. His lab has focused on gene therapy as a potential treatment for both hearing loss and dizziness. Gene therapy is an experimental technique that modifies a person's genes to treat a disease process.

Dr. Chien's colleagues at NIDCD have helped to characterize a mutation found in the "whirlin" gene. Mutations in this gene are associated with Usher syndrome, a condition that affects hearing and vision. Deafness resulting from the syndrome is caused by the abnormal development of hair cells in the inner ear. The syndrome also causes balance problems.

To test the effectiveness of gene therapy at treating balance problems and hearing loss, Dr. Chien delivered normal copies of "whirlin" cDNA to the inner ear of mice with a mutation affecting the "whirlin" gene, which causes these mutant mice to be deaf and to spin around. The hope is to replace the mutated gene with a healthy copy of the gene. He found that gene therapy treatment caused these mutant mice to have longer stereocilia—the hair-like projections on the hair cells—than mice that did not receive the gene therapy treatment. He found that the mutant mice that received gene therapy stopped spinning and started to walk in a straight line. In addition, he also found that these mutant mice could start to hear after gene therapy.

Dr. Chien said other researchers are also using gene-editing technologies, such as CRISPR-Cas9, to make changes in specific regions of the genome. In one study, Harvard University scientists prevented hearing loss in mice with hereditary deafness by using a gene-editing approach to disable a mutation that causes hearing loss. Research is ongoing.[1]

---

[1] "NIDCD Lab Applies Gene Therapy to Hearing Loss," National Institutes of Health (NIH), September 4, 2020. Available online. URL: https://nihrecord.nih.gov/2020/09/04/nidcd-lab-applies-gene-therapy-hearing-loss. Accessed October 9, 2024.

Part 5 | Assistive Hearing for People with Auditory Impairment

Chapter 15 | **Hearing Aids**

WHAT IS A HEARING AID?

A hearing aid is a small electronic device that one wears in or behind the ear. It makes some sounds louder so that a person with hearing loss can listen, communicate, and participate more fully in daily activities. A hearing aid can help people hear more in both quiet and noisy situations. However, only about one out of five people who would benefit from a hearing aid actually uses one.

A hearing aid has three basic parts: a microphone, an amplifier, and a speaker. The hearing aid receives sound through a microphone, which converts the sound waves to electrical signals and sends them to an amplifier. The amplifier increases the power of the signals and then sends them to the ear through a speaker.

HOW CAN HEARING AIDS HELP?

Hearing aids are primarily useful in improving the hearing and speech comprehension of people who have hearing loss resulting from damage to the small sensory cells in the inner ear, called "hair cells." This type of hearing loss is called "sensorineural hearing loss." The damage can occur as a result of disease, aging, or injury from noise or certain medicines.

A hearing aid magnifies sound vibrations entering the ear. Surviving hair cells detect the larger vibrations and convert them into neural signals that are passed along to the brain. The greater the damage to a person's hair cells, the more severe the hearing loss, and the greater the hearing aid amplification needed to make up the difference. However, there are practical limits to the amount of amplification a hearing aid can provide. In addition, if the inner ear is too damaged, even large vibrations will not be converted into neural signals. In this situation, a hearing aid would be ineffective.

WHERE CAN I GET HELP WITH MY HEARING LOSS?

If you or an adult family member have questions or concerns about hearing loss, there are options available. Over-the-counter (OTC) hearing aids are a new category of hearing aids that people can buy directly without visiting a hearing health professional for an examination. These hearing aids are intended to help adults with perceived mild to moderate hearing loss. Prescription hearing aids are available from a hearing health professional who will program them for your degree of hearing loss. Prescription hearing aids or other devices may be necessary for more significant or complicated hearing loss.

ARE THERE DIFFERENT STYLES OF HEARING AIDS?

There are three basic styles of hearing aids. The styles differ by size, placement on or inside the ear, and the degree to which they amplify sound (see Figure 15.1).

1. **Behind-the-ear (BTE) hearing aids.** They consist of a hard plastic case worn behind the ear and connected to a plastic earmold that fits inside the outer ear. The electronic parts are held in the case behind the ear. Sound travels from the hearing aid through the earmold and into the ear. BTE aids are used by people of all ages for mild to profound hearing loss. A new kind of BTE aid is the open-fit hearing aid. Small, open-fit aids fit behind the ear completely, with only a narrow tube inserted into the ear canal, enabling the canal to remain open. For this reason, open-fit hearing aids may be a good choice for people who experience a buildup of earwax since this type of aid is less likely to be damaged by such substances. In addition, some people may prefer the open-fit hearing aid because their perception of their voice does not sound "plugged up."

2. **In-the-ear (ITE) hearing aids.** They fit completely inside the outer ear and are used for mild to severe hearing loss. The case holding the electronic components is made of hard plastic. Some ITE aids may have certain added features installed, such as a telecoil. A telecoil is a small magnetic coil that allows users to receive sound through the circuitry of the hearing aid rather than through its microphone.

Hearing Aids | 163

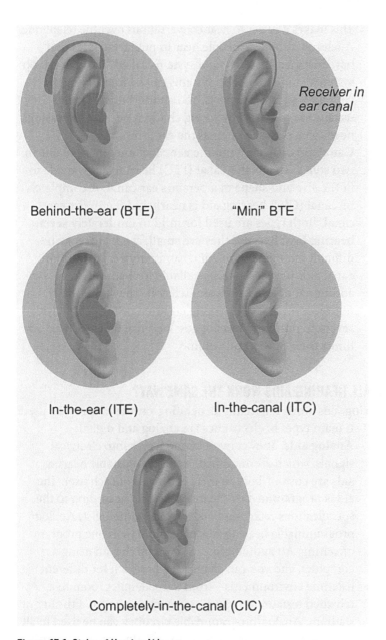

Figure 15.1. Styles of Hearing Aids
National Institute on Deafness and Other Communication Disorders (NIDCD)

This makes it easier to hear conversations over the telephone. A telecoil also helps people hear in public facilities that have installed special sound systems called "induction loop systems." Induction loop systems can be found in many churches, schools, airports, and auditoriums. ITE aids usually are not worn by young children because the casings need to be replaced often as the ear grows.
3. **Canal aids.** They fit into the ear canal and are available in two styles. The in-the-canal (ITC) hearing aid is made to fit the size and shape of a person's ear canal. A completely-in-canal (CIC) hearing aid is nearly hidden in the ear canal. Both types are used for mild to moderately severe hearing loss. Because they are small, canal aids may be difficult for a person to adjust and remove. In addition, canal aids have less space available for batteries and additional devices, such as a telecoil. They are usually not recommended for young children or for people with severe to profound hearing loss because their reduced size limits their power and volume.

DO ALL HEARING AIDS WORK THE SAME WAY?
Hearing aids work differently depending on the electronics used. The two main types of electronics are analog and digital.
1. **Analog aids.** They convert sound waves into electrical signals, which are amplified. Analog/adjustable hearing aids are custom-built to meet the needs of each user. The aid is programmed by the manufacturer according to the specifications recommended by your audiologist. Analog/programmable hearing aids have more than one program or setting. An audiologist can program the aid using a computer, and you can change the program for different listening environments—from a small, quiet room to a crowded restaurant to large, open areas, such as a theater or stadium. Analog/programmable circuitry can be used in all types of hearing aids. Analog aids usually are less expensive than digital aids.

2. **Digital aids**. They convert sound waves into numerical codes, similar to the binary code of a computer, before amplifying them. Because the code also includes information about a sound's pitch or loudness, the aid can be specially programmed to amplify some frequencies more than others. Digital circuitry gives an audiologist more flexibility in adjusting the aid to a user's needs and to certain listening environments. These aids also can be programmed to focus on sounds coming from a specific direction. Digital circuitry can be used in all types of hearing aids.

HOW CAN I ADJUST TO MY HEARING AID?

Hearing aids take time and patience to use successfully. Wearing your aids regularly will help you adjust to them.

Become familiar with your hearing aid's features. With your audiologist present, practice putting in and taking out the aid, cleaning it, identifying right and left aids, and replacing the batteries. Ask how to test it in listening environments where you have problems hearing. Learn to adjust the aid's volume and to program it for sounds that are too loud or too soft. Work with your audiologist until you are comfortable and satisfied.

You may experience some of the following problems as you adjust to wearing your new aid:

- **My hearing aid feels uncomfortable**. Some individuals may find hearing aids slightly uncomfortable at first. Ask your audiologist how long you should wear them while you are adjusting to them.
- **My voice sounds too loud**. The "plugged-up" sensation that causes a hearing aid user's voice to sound louder inside the head is called the "occlusion effect," and it is very common for new hearing aid users. Check with your audiologist to see if a correction is possible. Most individuals get used to this effect over time.
- **I get feedback from my hearing aid**. A whistling sound can be caused by a hearing aid that does not fit or work

well or is clogged by earwax or fluid. See your audiologist for adjustments.
- **I hear background noise**. A hearing aid does not completely separate the sounds you want to hear from the ones you do not want to hear. Sometimes, however, the hearing aid may need to be adjusted. Talk with your audiologist.
- **I hear a buzzing sound when I use my cell phone**. Some people who wear hearing aids or have implanted hearing devices experience problems with the radio frequency interference caused by digital cell phones. However, both hearing aids and cell phones are improving, so these problems are occurring less often. When you are being fitted for a new hearing aid, take your cell phone with you to see if it will work well with the aid.

HOW CAN I CARE FOR MY HEARING AID?

Proper maintenance and care will extend the life of your hearing aid. Make it a habit to take the following actions:
- Keep hearing aids away from heat and moisture.
- Clean hearing aids as instructed. Earwax and ear drainage can damage a hearing aid.
- Avoid using hairspray or other hair care products while wearing hearing aids.
- Turn off hearing aids when they are not in use.
- Replace dead batteries immediately.
- Keep replacement batteries and small aids away from children and pets.[1]

---

[1] "Hearing Aids," National Institute on Deafness and Other Communication Disorders (NIDCD), October 11, 2022. Available online. URL: www.nidcd.nih.gov/health/hearing-aids. Accessed October 10, 2024.

Chapter 16 | **Over-the-Counter Hearing Aids**

UNDERSTANDING OVER-THE-COUNTER HEARING AIDS
Over-the-counter (OTC) hearing aids are a new category of hearing aids that consumers can purchase directly without visiting a hearing health professional. These devices are intended to help adults with perceived mild to moderate hearing loss. Like prescription hearing aids, OTC hearing aids amplify sounds, enabling some adults with difficulty hearing to better listen, communicate, and participate fully in daily activities. Additionally, the U.S. Food and Drug Administration (FDA) regulates OTC hearing aids as medical devices.

COMPARISON WITH PRESCRIPTION HEARING AIDS
Over-the-counter hearing aids are an alternative to prescription hearing aids, which are currently only available from hearing health professionals, such as audiologists, otolaryngologists (ear, nose, and throat doctors), and hearing aid specialists. Hearing health professionals fit individuals for hearing aids, adjust the devices based on hearing loss, and provide other services.

ACCESSIBILITY AND USER CONTROL
Consumers can now buy OTC hearing aids directly in stores and online. Users fit them themselves and may be able to control and adjust the devices in ways that users of prescription hearing aids cannot. Some OTC hearing aids might not resemble prescription hearing aids at all.

INTENDED USE AND LIMITATIONS
Over-the-counter hearing aids are designed for adults with perceived mild to moderate hearing loss. They are not intended for

children or for adults who have more severe hearing loss or significant difficulty hearing. If an individual has more severe hearing loss, OTC hearing aids might not amplify sounds at high enough levels to be effective.

REGULATORY STANDARDS AND CONSUMER GUIDANCE

The FDA has established regulations that manufacturers of OTC hearing aids must follow. In general, these federal regulations are designed to:
- Ensure that OTC devices are safe and effective for people with perceived mild to moderate hearing loss.
- Set standards for package labels to help buyers understand OTC hearing aids and identify who might benefit from them. The labels also include warnings and other information consumers should know before purchasing or using the hearing aid, such as signs that indicate a need to see a doctor.

PERSONAL SOUND AMPLIFICATION PRODUCTS

Personal sound amplification products (PSAPs) are another class of amplifying devices that can be purchased without a prescription or consulting a health-care professional. They are intended for people without hearing loss and enhance the ability to hear certain sounds in specific situations, such as bird-watching. While the FDA regulates OTC hearing aids as medical devices for adults with hearing loss, PSAPs are not regulated as medical devices by the FDA.

WHO SHOULD CONSIDER OTC HEARING AIDS?

Over-the-counter hearing aids are for adults (18 and older) who believe they have mild to moderate hearing loss, even if they have not had a hearing exam. Indicators of mild to moderate hearing loss may include the following:
- Speech or other sounds seem muffled.
- Difficulty hearing in groups, in noisy areas, on the phone, or when unable to see the speaker.
- Needing to ask others to speak more slowly or clearly, talk louder, or repeat what they said.

- Turning up the volume higher than others prefer when watching TV or listening to the radio or music.
- People with hearing difficulties may have trouble hearing conversations in quiet settings or difficulty hearing loud sounds, such as cars or trucks, noisy appliances, or loud music.

If experiencing trouble hearing conversations in quiet settings or loud sounds, consult a hearing health professional. These signs may indicate more severe hearing loss, and OTC hearing aids may not be effective. A hearing health professional can help determine if a prescription hearing aid or another device can improve hearing.

WHEN TO SEEK MEDICAL ATTENTION

Certain ear problems require medical treatment. If experiencing any of the following, see a licensed physician promptly:
- fluid, pus, or blood coming out of the ear within the previous six months
- pain or discomfort in the ear
- a history of excessive earwax or suspicion that something is in the ear canal
- episodes of vertigo (severe dizziness) with hearing loss
- sudden or rapidly worsening hearing loss
- hearing loss that fluctuates in severity within the last six months
- hearing loss or tinnitus (ringing) in only one ear, or a noticeable difference in hearing between ears

THE EFFECT OF HEARING LOSS ON QUALITY OF LIFE

Hearing loss significantly affects the quality of life for tens of millions of adults in the United States and contributes to high healthcare costs. Untreated hearing loss can lead to isolation and has been associated with serious conditions such as:
- depression
- anxiety
- low self-esteem

- dementia
- reduced mobility
- falls

Despite these consequences, only one in four adults who could benefit from hearing aids has ever used them. Making hearing health care more accessible and affordable is a public health priority, especially as the number of older adults in the United States continues to grow.

COLLABORATIVE EFFORTS TO IMPROVE HEARING HEALTHCARE ACCESS

Leading experts in science, technology, and hearing health care have collaborated with researchers, health professionals, and consumers to find safe and effective ways to improve access to hearing health care for adults. They suggested changing some regulations that studies showed were barriers to adults obtaining the hearing help they need. They also recommended that the FDA create guidelines and quality standards for OTC hearing aids.

As the FDA continues to regulate and refine OTC hearing aids, they provide a valuable alternative to traditional prescription hearing aids, expanding options for those seeking to enhance their hearing capabilities.[1]

---

[1] "Over-the-Counter Hearing Aids," National Institute on Deafness and Other Communication Disorders (NIDCD), June 13, 2024. Available online. URL: www.nidcd.nih.gov/health/over-counter-hearing-aids. Accessed October 9, 2024.

Chapter 17 | Cochlear Implants

WHAT IS A COCHLEAR IMPLANT?
A cochlear implant is a small, complex electronic device that can help provide a sense of sound to a person who is profoundly deaf or severely hard of hearing. The implant consists of an external portion that sits behind the ear and a second portion that is surgically placed under the skin.

An implant has the following parts:
- **Microphone**. Picks up sound from the environment.
- **Speech processor**. Selects and arranges sounds picked up by the microphone.
- **Transmitter and receiver/stimulator**. Receive signals from the speech processor and convert them into electric impulses.
- **Electrode array**. A group of electrodes that collects the impulses from the stimulator and sends them to different regions of the auditory nerve.

An implant does not restore normal hearing. Instead, it can provide a person with deafness a useful representation of sounds in the environment and assist in understanding speech.

HOW DOES A COCHLEAR IMPLANT WORK?
A cochlear implant is fundamentally different from a hearing aid. While hearing aids amplify sounds so they may be detected by damaged ears, cochlear implants bypass damaged portions of the ear and directly stimulate the auditory nerve. Signals generated by the implant are sent via the auditory nerve to the brain, which recognizes the signals as sound. Hearing through a cochlear implant is different from normal hearing and takes time to learn or relearn. However, it allows many people to recognize warning signals,

understand other sounds in the environment, and comprehend speech in person or over the telephone.

WHO GETS COCHLEAR IMPLANTS?

Children and adults who are deaf or severely hard of hearing can be fitted for cochlear implants. As of December 2019, approximately 736,900 registered devices have been implanted worldwide. In the United States, roughly 118,100 devices have been implanted in adults and 65,000 in children (estimates provided by the U.S. Food and Drug Administration (FDA), as reported by cochlear implant manufacturers approved for the U.S. market).

- **Children.** The FDA first approved cochlear implants in the mid-1980s to treat hearing loss in adults. Since 2020, cochlear implants have been FDA approved for use in eligible children beginning at nine months of age. For young children who are deaf or severely hard of hearing, using a cochlear implant early exposes them to sounds during an optimal period to develop speech and language skills. Research has shown that when children receive a cochlear implant early in life followed by intensive therapy, they are often better able to hear, comprehend sound and music, and speak than their peers who receive implants when they are older. Studies have also demonstrated that eligible children (as young as 9 months of age) who receive a cochlear implant early may develop language skills at a rate comparable to children with normal hearing and many succeed in mainstream classrooms.
- **Adults.** Some adults who have lost all or most of their hearing later in life can also benefit from cochlear implants. They learn to associate the signals from the implant with sounds they remember, including speech, without requiring any visual cues such as those provided by lipreading or sign language.

HOW DOES SOMEONE RECEIVE A COCHLEAR IMPLANT?

Receiving a cochlear implant involves both a surgical procedure and significant therapy to learn or relearn the sense of hearing. Not everyone performs at the same level with this device. The decision to receive an implant should involve discussions with medical specialists, including an experienced cochlear-implant surgeon. The process can be expensive; for example, a person's health insurance may cover the expense, but not always. Some individuals may choose not to have a cochlear implant for a variety of personal reasons.

Considerations
- **Safety**. Surgical implantations are almost always safe, although complications are a risk factor, as with any kind of surgery.
- **Learning curve**. Learning to interpret the sounds created by an implant takes time and practice. Speech-language pathologists (SLPs) and audiologists are frequently involved in this learning process.
- **Assessment**. All factors, including medical suitability, potential benefits, and personal considerations, need to be thoroughly assessed prior to implantation.[1]

---

[1] "Cochlear Implants," National Institute on Deafness and Other Communication Disorders (NIDCD), June 13, 2024. Available online. URL: www.nidcd.nih.gov/health/cochlear-implants. Accessed October 9, 2024.

Chapter 18 | **Assistive Devices for Hearing Loss**

WHAT ARE ASSISTIVE DEVICES?
The terms "assistive device" or "assistive technology" can refer to any device that helps a person with hearing loss or a voice, speech, or language disorder to communicate. These terms often refer to devices that help a person hear and understand what is being said more clearly or express thoughts more easily. With the development of digital and wireless technologies, more and more devices are becoming available to help people with hearing, voice, speech, and language disorders communicate more meaningfully and participate more fully in their daily lives.

WHAT TYPES OF ASSISTIVE DEVICES ARE AVAILABLE?
Health professionals use a variety of names to describe assistive devices:
- **Assistive listening devices (ALDs).** They amplify sounds you want to hear, especially where there is a lot of background noise. ALDs can be used with a hearing aid or cochlear implant to help a wearer hear certain sounds better.
- **Augmentative and alternative communication (AAC) devices.** These devices help people with communication disorders express themselves. They can range from a simple picture board to a computer program that synthesizes speech from text.
- **Alerting devices.** They connect to a doorbell, telephone, or alarm that emits a loud sound or blinking light to let someone with hearing loss know that an event is taking place.

WHAT TYPES OF ASSISTIVE LISTENING DEVICES ARE AVAILABLE?

Several types of ALDs are available to improve sound transmission for people with hearing loss. Some are designed for large facilities such as classrooms, theaters, places of worship, and airports. Other types are intended for personal use in small settings and for one-on-one conversations. All can be used with or without hearing aids or a cochlear implant. ALD systems for large facilities include hearing loop systems, frequency-modulated (FM) systems, and infrared systems.

- **Hearing loop (or induction loop) systems use electromagnetic energy to transmit sound.** A hearing loop system involves four parts:
  1. a sound source, such as a public address system, microphone, or home TV or telephone
  2. an amplifier
  3. a thin loop of wire that encircles a room or branches out beneath carpeting
  4. a receiver worn in the ears or as a headset

Amplified sound travels through the loop and creates an electromagnetic field that is picked up directly by a hearing loop receiver or a telecoil. A telecoil is a coil of wire installed inside many hearing aids and cochlear implants that acts as a miniature wireless receiver. To pick up the signal, a listener must be wearing the receiver and be within or near the loop. Because the sound is picked up directly by the receiver, the sound is much clearer, without as much of the competing background noise associated with many listening environments. Some loop systems are portable, making it possible for people with hearing loss to improve their listening environments, as needed, as they proceed with their daily activities. A hearing loop can be connected to a public address system, a television, or any other audio source. For those who do not have hearing aids with embedded telecoils, portable loop receivers are also available.

- **FM systems use radio signals to transmit amplified sounds.** They are often used in classrooms, where the instructor wears a small microphone connected to a transmitter, and the student wears the receiver, which is tuned to a specific frequency or channel. People who have a telecoil inside their hearing aid or cochlear implant may also wear a wire around the neck (called a "neckloop") or behind their aid or implant (called a "silhouette inductor") to convert the signal into magnetic signals that can be picked up directly by the telecoil. FM systems can transmit signals up to 300 feet and are able to be used in many public places. However, because radio signals can penetrate walls, listeners in one room may need to listen to a different channel than those in another room to avoid receiving mixed signals. Personal FM systems operate in the same way as larger scale systems and can be used to help people with hearing loss follow one-on-one conversations.

- **Infrared systems use infrared light to transmit sound.** A transmitter converts sound into a light signal and beams it to a receiver that is worn by a listener. The receiver decodes the infrared signal back to sound. As with FM systems, people whose hearing aids or cochlear implants have a telecoil may also wear a neckloop or silhouette inductor to convert the infrared signal into a magnetic signal, which can be picked up through their telecoil. Unlike induction loop or FM systems, the infrared signal cannot pass through walls, making it particularly useful in courtrooms, where confidential information is often discussed, and in buildings where competing signals can be a problem, such as classrooms or movie theaters. However, infrared systems cannot be used in environments with too many competing light sources, such as outdoors or in strongly lit rooms.
- **Personal amplifiers are useful in places where the above systems are unavailable or when watching TV, being outdoors, or traveling in a car.** About the size of a cell phone, these devices increase sound levels and reduce background noise for a listener. Some have directional microphones that can be angled toward a speaker or other source of sound. As with other ALDs, the amplified sound can be picked up by a receiver that the listener is wearing, either as a headset or as earbuds.

WHAT TYPES OF AUGMENTATIVE AND ALTERNATIVE COMMUNICATION DEVICES ARE AVAILABLE FOR COMMUNICATING FACE-TO-FACE?

The simplest AAC device is a picture board or touch screen that uses pictures or symbols of typical items and activities that make up a person's daily life. For example, a person might touch the image of a glass to ask for a drink. Many picture boards can be customized and expanded based on a person's age, education, occupation, and interests.

Keyboards, touch screens, and sometimes a person's limited speech may be used to communicate desired words. Some devices employ a text display. The display panel typically faces outward so that two people can exchange information while facing each other. Spelling and word prediction software can make it faster and easier to enter information.

Speech-generating devices go one step further by translating words or pictures into speech. Some models allow users to choose from several different voices, such as male or female, child or adult, and even some regional accents. Some devices employ a vocabulary of prerecorded words while others have an unlimited vocabulary, synthesizing speech as words are typed in. Software programs that convert personal computers into speaking devices are also available.

WHAT AUGMENTATIVE AND ALTERNATIVE COMMUNICATION DEVICES ARE AVAILABLE FOR COMMUNICATING BY TELEPHONE?

For many years, people with hearing loss have used text telephone or telecommunications devices, called "TTY or TDD machines," to communicate by phone. This same technology also benefits people with speech difficulties. A TTY machine consists of a typewriter keyboard that displays typed conversations onto a readout panel or printed on paper. Callers will either type messages to each other over the system or, if a call recipient does not have a TTY machine, use the national toll-free telecommunications relay service at 711 to communicate (www.nidcd.nih.gov/health/telecomm). Through the relay service, a communications assistant serves as a bridge between two callers, reading typed messages aloud to the person

Assistive Devices for Hearing Loss | 179

with hearing while transcribing what is spoken into type for the person with hearing loss.

With today's new electronic communication devices, however, TTY machines have almost become a thing of the past. People can place phone calls through the telecommunications relay service using almost any device with a keypad, including a laptop, personal digital assistant, and cell phone. Text messaging has also become a popular method of communication, skipping the relay service altogether.

Another system uses voice recognition software and an extensive library of video clips depicting American Sign Language to translate a signer's words into text or computer-generated speech in real time. It is also able to translate spoken words back into sign language or text.

Finally, for people with mild to moderate hearing loss, captioned telephones allow you to carry on a spoken conversation while providing a transcript of the other person's words on a readout panel or computer screen as backup.

WHAT TYPES OF ALERTING DEVICES ARE AVAILABLE?

Alerting or alarm devices use sound, light, vibrations, or a combination of these techniques to let someone know when a particular event is occurring. Clocks and wake-up alarm systems allow a person to choose to wake up to flashing lights, horns, or a gentle shaking.

Visual alert signalers monitor a variety of household devices and other sounds, such as doorbells and telephones. When the phone rings, the visual alert signaler will be activated and will vibrate or flash a light to let people know. In addition, remote receivers placed around the house can alert a person from any room. Portable vibrating pagers can let parents and caretakers know when a baby is crying. Some baby monitoring devices analyze a baby's cry and light up a picture to indicate if the baby sounds hungry, bored, or sleepy.[1]

---

[1] "Assistive Devices for People with Hearing, Voice, Speech, or Language Disorders," National Institute on Deafness and Other Communication Disorders (NIDCD), November 12, 2019. Available online. URL: www.nidcd.nih.gov/health/assistive-devices-people-hearing-voice-speech-or-language-disorders. Accessed October 10, 2024.

Chapter 19 | Captioning and Visual Tools for Viewers with Hearing Impairments

WHAT ARE CAPTIONS?

Captions are words displayed on a television, computer, mobile device, or movie screen that describe the audio or sound portion of a program or video. Captions allow viewers who are deaf or hard of hearing to follow the dialogue and the action of a program simultaneously. For people with hearing loss who are not deaf, captions can even make the spoken words easier to hear—because hearing, like vision, is influenced by our expectations. For example, when you have an idea of what someone might be about to say, their speech may seem clearer. Captions can also provide information about who is speaking or about sound effects that may be important to understanding a news story, a political event, or the plot of a program.

HOW ARE CAPTIONS CREATED?

Captions are created from the program's transcript. A captioner separates the dialogue into captions and ensures the words appear in sync with the audio they describe. Computer software encodes the captioning information and combines it with the audio and video to create a new master tape or digital file of the program. Ideally, captions should appear near the bottom of the screen—not in the middle, where misplaced captions can cover important visuals such as a newscaster's face or a basketball hoop.

TYPES OF CAPTIONS
Open and Closed Captions
- **Open captions.** Always visible and cannot be turned off.
- **Closed captions.** Can be turned on and off by the viewer using the menu settings on any television.

Closed captioning is available on digital television sets, including high-definition televisions manufactured after July 1, 2002. Some digital captioning menus allow viewers to control the caption display, including font style, text size and color, and background color.

Real-Time Captioning
Real-time captions, or communication access real-time translation, are created as an event takes place. A captioner (often trained as a court reporter or stenographer) uses a stenotype machine with a phonetic keyboard and special software. A computer translates the phonetic symbols into English captions almost instantaneously. Real-time captioning can be used for programs that have no script, live events (including congressional proceedings), news programs, and non-broadcast meetings such as the national meetings of professional associations.

Electronic Newsroom Captions
Electronic newsroom captions (ENR) are created from a news script computer or teleprompter and are commonly used for live newscasts. This technique can caption only scripted material. Therefore, spontaneous commentary, live field reports, breaking news, and sports and weather updates may not be captioned using ENR, necessitating real-time captioning for those segments.

Edited and Verbatim Captions
- **Edited captions.** Summarize ideas and shorten phrases for ease of reading, often preferred for children's programs.
- **Verbatim captions.** Include all spoken words, providing full access and detailed information preferred by most people who are deaf or hard of hearing.

Rear-Window Captioning
Some movie theaters offer this captioning system. An adjustable Lucite panel attaches to the viewer's seat and reflects the captions from a light-emitting diode (LED) panel at the back of the theater.

Captioned Telephone
A captioned telephone has a built-in screen to display text (captions) of whatever the other person on the call is saying. When an outgoing call is placed on a captioned telephone, the call is connected to a Captioned Telephone Service (CTS). A specially trained CTS operator hears the person you want to talk to and repeats what that person says. Speech recognition technology automatically transcribes the CTS operator's voice into text displayed on the captioned telephone screen.

THE LAW AND CAPTIONING
Americans with Disabilities Act of 1990
The Americans with Disabilities Act (ADA) of 1990 requires businesses and public accommodations to ensure that individuals with disabilities are not excluded from or denied services because of the absence of auxiliary aids. Captions are considered one type of auxiliary aid. Since the passage of the ADA, the use of captioning has expanded significantly. Entertainment, educational, informational, and training materials are captioned for deaf and hard of hearing audiences at the time they are produced and distributed.

Television Decoder Circuitry Act of 1990
The Television Decoder Circuitry Act of 1990 requires that all televisions larger than 13 inches sold in the United States after July 1993 have a special built-in decoder that enables viewers to watch closed-captioned programming.

Telecommunications Act of 1996
The Telecommunications Act of 1996 directs the Federal Communications Commission (FCC) to adopt rules requiring closed captioning of most television programming.

FCC Rules on Closed Captioning

Effective January 1, 1998, the FCC's rules require people or companies that distribute television programs directly to home viewers to caption those programs. By January 1, 2006, all non-exempt programs were required to be closed-captioned, and after that date, captioning was also required for all new non-exempt programs. As of January 1, 2010, all new non-exempt Spanish-language video programming must also be provided with captions. Detailed guidelines and definitions of terms are available in the FCC's Electronic Code of Federal Regulations (www.fcc.gov/general/closed-captioning-video-programming-television).

Who Must Provide Closed Captions?

Congress requires video program distributors (cable operators, broadcasters, satellite distributors, and other multichannel video programming distributors) to close caption their TV programs. FCC rules ensure that viewers have full access to programming, address captioning quality, and provide guidance to video programming distributors and programmers. The rules require that captions be accurate, synchronous, complete, and properly placed. They distinguish between prerecorded, live, and near-live programming, recognizing the greater challenges involved with captioning live or near-live programming.

Exempt Programs

Some advertisements, public service announcements, non-English-language programs (except Spanish programs), locally produced and distributed non-news programming, textual programs, early-morning programs, and nonvocal musical programs are exempt from captioning.

HOW TO ACCESS MORE INFORMATION

To find out more about the FCC rules and captions, including information on the complaint process, you can contact:
- Toll-free voice: 888-CALL-FCC (888-225-5322).
- ASL video call: 844-432-2275.
- Fax: 866-418-0232.

Captioning and Visual Tools for Viewers with Hearing Impairments

As technology continues to advance, captions will remain a vital component of inclusive media consumption, promoting equal access and enhancing the viewing experience for all.[1]

---

[1] "Captions for Deaf and Hard-of-Hearing Viewers," National Institute on Deafness and Other Communication Disorders (NIDCD), July 5, 2017. Available online. URL: www.nidcd.nih.gov/health/captions-deaf-and-hard-hearing-viewers. Accessed October 9, 2024.

Part 6 | Disability Rights for Auditory Impairment

Chapter 20 | Legal Protections for People with Auditory Impairments

AMERICANS WITH DISABILITIES ACT

The Americans with Disabilities Act (ADA) prohibits discrimination on the basis of disability in employment, state and local government, public accommodations, commercial facilities, transportation, and telecommunications.

To be protected by the ADA, one must have a disability or have a relationship or association with an individual with a disability. An individual with a disability is defined by the ADA as a person who has a physical or mental impairment that substantially limits one or more major life activities, a person who has a history or record of such an impairment, or a person who is perceived by others as having such an impairment. The ADA does not specifically name all the impairments that are covered.

ADA Title II: State and Local Government Activities

Title II covers all activities of state and local governments regardless of the government entity's size or receipt of federal funding. Title II requires that state and local governments give people with disabilities an equal opportunity to benefit from all of their programs, services, and activities (e.g., public education, employment, transportation, recreation, health care, social services, courts, voting, and town meetings).

State and local governments are required to follow specific architectural standards in the new construction and alteration of their buildings. They must also relocate programs or otherwise provide access in inaccessible older buildings, and communicate effectively with people who have hearing, vision, or speech disabilities. Public entities are not required to take actions that would result in undue financial and administrative burdens. They are required to make reasonable modifications to policies, practices, and procedures where necessary to avoid discrimination, unless they can demonstrate that doing so would fundamentally alter the nature of the service, program, or activity being provided.

ADA Title III: Public Accommodations

Title III covers businesses and nonprofit service providers that are public accommodations, privately operated entities offering certain types of courses and examinations, privately operated transportation, and commercial facilities. Public accommodations are private entities that own, lease, lease to, or operate facilities such as restaurants, retail stores, hotels, movie theaters, private schools, convention centers, doctors' offices, homeless shelters, transportation depots, zoos, funeral homes, day care centers, and recreation facilities including sports stadiums and fitness clubs. Transportation services provided by private entities are also covered by Title III.

Public accommodations must comply with basic nondiscrimination requirements that prohibit exclusion, segregation, and unequal treatment. They also must comply with specific requirements related to architectural standards for new and altered buildings; reasonable modifications to policies, practices, and procedures; effective communication with people with hearing, vision, or speech disabilities; and other access requirements. Additionally, public accommodations must remove barriers in existing buildings where it is easy to do so without much difficulty or expense, given the public accommodation's resources.

Courses and examinations related to professional, educational, or trade-related applications, licensing, certifications, or credentialing must be provided in a place and manner accessible to people with disabilities, or alternative accessible arrangements must be offered.

Commercial facilities, such as factories and warehouses, must comply with the ADA's architectural standards for new construction and alterations.

ADA Title IV: Telecommunications Relay Services

Title IV addresses telephone and television access for people with hearing and speech disabilities. It requires common carriers (telephone companies) to establish interstate and intrastate telecommunications relay services (TRS) 24 hours a day, 7 days a week. TRS enables callers with hearing and speech disabilities who use TTYs (also known as "TDDs") and callers who use voice telephones to communicate with each other through a third-party communications assistant. The Federal Communications Commission (FCC) has set minimum standards for TRS services. Title IV also requires closed captioning of federally funded public service announcements.

TELECOMMUNICATIONS ACT

Section 255 and Section 251(a)(2) of the Communications Act of 1934, as amended by the Telecommunications Act of 1996, require manufacturers of telecommunications equipment and providers of telecommunications services to ensure that such equipment and services are accessible to and usable by people with disabilities, if readily achievable. These amendments ensure that people with disabilities will have access to a broad range of products and services such as telephones, cell phones, pagers, call-waiting, and operator services, which were often inaccessible to many users with disabilities.

FAIR HOUSING ACT

The Fair Housing Act, as amended in 1988, prohibits housing discrimination on the basis of race, color, religion, sex, disability, familial status, and national origin. Its coverage includes private housing, housing that receives federal financial assistance, and state and local government housing. It is unlawful to discriminate in any aspect of selling or renting housing or to deny a dwelling to a buyer or renter because of the disability of that individual, an individual associated with the buyer or renter, or an individual who intends to live in the residence. Other covered activities include, for example, financing, zoning practices, new construction design, and advertising.

The Fair Housing Act requires owners of housing facilities to make reasonable exceptions in their policies and operations to afford people with disabilities equal housing opportunities. For example, a landlord with a "no pets" policy may be required to grant an exception to this rule and allow an individual who is blind to keep a guide dog in the residence. The Fair Housing Act also requires landlords to allow tenants with disabilities to make reasonable access-related modifications to their private living space, as well as to common-use spaces. (The landlord is not required to pay for the changes.) The Act further requires that new multi-family housing with four or more units be designed and built to allow access for people with disabilities. This includes accessible common-use areas, doors that are wide enough for wheelchairs, kitchens, and bathrooms that allow a person using a wheelchair to maneuver, and other adaptable features within the units.

INDIVIDUALS WITH DISABILITIES EDUCATION ACT

The Individuals with Disabilities Education Act (IDEA) requires public schools to provide all eligible children with disabilities with a free, appropriate public education in the least restrictive environment appropriate to their individual needs.

IDEA requires public school systems to develop appropriate Individualized Education Programs (IEPs) for each child. The specific special education and related services outlined in each IEP reflect the individualized needs of each student.

IDEA also mandates that particular procedures be followed in the development of the IEP. Each student's IEP must be developed by a team of knowledgeable people and must be at least reviewed annually. The team includes the child's teacher; the parents, subject to certain limited exceptions; the child, if determined appropriate; an agency representative who is qualified to provide or supervise the provision of special education; and other individuals at the parents' or agency's discretion.

REHABILITATION ACT

The Rehabilitation Act prohibits discrimination on the basis of disability in programs conducted by federal agencies, in programs receiving federal financial assistance, in federal employment, and in the employment practices of federal contractors. The standards for determining employment discrimination under the Rehabilitation Act are the same as those used in Title I of the Americans With Disabilities Act.

Section 504

Section 504 states that "no qualified individual with a disability in the United States shall be excluded from, denied the benefits of, or be subjected to discrimination under" any program or activity that either receives federal financial assistance or is conducted by any executive agency or the United States Postal Service.

Each federal agency has its own set of Section 504 regulations that apply to its own programs. Agencies that provide federal financial assistance also have Section 504 regulations covering entities that receive federal aid. Requirements common to these regulations include reasonable accommodation for employees with disabilities; program accessibility; effective communication with people who have hearing or vision disabilities; and accessible new construction and alterations. Each agency is responsible for enforcing its own regulations. Section 504 may also be enforced through private lawsuits. It is not necessary to file a complaint with a federal agency or to receive a "right-to-sue" letter before going to court.

Section 508

Section 508 establishes requirements for electronic and information technology developed, maintained, procured, or used by the federal government. Section 508 requires federal electronic and information technology to be accessible to people with disabilities, including employees and members of the public.

An accessible information technology system is one that can be operated in various ways and does not rely on a single sense or ability of the user. For example, a system that provides output only in visual format may not be accessible to people with visual impairments, and a system that provides output only in audio format may not be accessible to people who are deaf or hard of hearing. Some people with disabilities may need accessibility-related software or peripheral devices in order to use systems that comply with Section 508.[1]

---

[1] ADA.gov, "Guide to Disability Rights Laws," U.S. Department of Justice (DOJ), February 28, 2020. Available online. URL: www.ada.gov/resources/disability-rights-guide. Accessed October 10, 2024.

Chapter 21 | Hearing Impairments and Employment Rights

Approximately 15 percent of American adults report some trouble hearing. There are many different circumstances that may contribute to people becoming deaf, hard of hearing, or experiencing other hearing conditions (including childhood illnesses, pregnancy-related illnesses, injury, heredity, age, and excessive or prolonged exposure to noise). These circumstances can affect the way such people experience sound, communicate with others, and view their hearing conditions. For example, some people who develop a hearing condition later in life may not use "American Sign Language" (ASL) or other common communication methods used by some with hearing conditions or may not use them as proficiently as some people who are deaf or hard of hearing from birth or a very young age.

People who are deaf, hard of hearing, or have other hearing conditions can perform successfully on the job and, under the Americans with Disabilities Act (ADA), should not be denied opportunities because of stereotypical assumptions about those conditions. Some employers assume incorrectly that workers with hearing conditions will cause safety hazards, increase employment costs, or have difficulty communicating in fast-paced environments. In reality, with or without reasonable accommodation, people with hearing conditions can be effective and safe workers.

HEARING CONDITION AS A DISABILITY UNDER THE ADA
According to the ADA, the definition of "disability" is interpreted broadly in favor of expansive coverage. Under the ADA, people

with an impairment of hearing will meet the first prong of the ADA's definition of disability (actual disability) if they can show that they are substantially limited in hearing or another major life activity (e.g., the major bodily function of special sense organs). A determination of disability must ignore the positive effects of any mitigating measure that is used. For example, if someone uses a hearing aid or has a cochlear implant, the benefits of such a device would not be considered when determining if the impairment is substantially limiting. People who are deaf should easily be found to have a disability within the meaning of the first part of the ADA's definition of disability because they are substantially limited in the major life activity of hearing.

People with a history of an impairment will be covered under the second prong of the ADA definition of disability if they have a record of an impairment that substantially limited a major life activity in the past. An applicant or employee may have a "record of" disability, for example, when the person's hearing has been corrected surgically. Finally, a person is covered under the third (regarded as) prong of the ADA definition of disability if an employer takes a prohibited action (i.e., refuses to hire or terminates the person) because of a hearing condition or because the employer believes the person has an impairment of hearing, other than an impairment that is not both transitory and minor.

MAY AN EMPLOYER ASK WHETHER A JOB APPLICANT HAS OR HAD A HEARING CONDITION, OR TREATMENT RELATED TO A HEARING CONDITION, PRIOR TO MAKING A JOB OFFER?

No. An employer may not ask questions about an applicant's medical condition or require an applicant to have a medical examination before they make a conditional job offer. This means that an employer cannot ask an applicant such questions as:
- whether the applicant has ever had any medical procedures related to hearing (i.e., whether the applicant has a cochlear implant)
- whether the applicant uses a hearing aid
- whether the applicant has any condition that affects the applicant's hearing

Of course, an employer may ask questions pertaining to the applicant's ability to perform the essential functions of the position, with or without reasonable accommodation, such as:
- whether the applicant can respond quickly to instructions in a noisy, fast-paced work environment
- whether the applicant has good communication skills
- whether the applicant can meet legally mandated safety standards required to perform a job

DOES THE ADA REQUIRE AN APPLICANT TO DISCLOSE A CURRENT OR PAST DISABILITY BEFORE ACCEPTING A JOB OFFER?

No. The ADA does not require applicants to disclose that they have or had a hearing disability or another disability unless they will need a reasonable accommodation for the application process (i.e., a sign language interpreter). Some people with a hearing condition, however, choose to disclose or discuss their condition to dispel myths about it or to ensure that employers do not assume that the condition means the person is unable to do the job.

Sometimes, the decision to disclose depends on whether a person will need a reasonable accommodation to perform the job (i.e., specialized equipment, removal of a marginal function, or another type of job restructuring). A person with a hearing condition, however, may request an accommodation after becoming an employee even if they did not do so when applying for the job or after receiving the job offer.

MAY AN EMPLOYER ASK QUESTIONS ABOUT AN OBVIOUS HEARING CONDITION, OR ASK FOLLOW-UP QUESTIONS IF AN APPLICANT DISCLOSES A NON-OBVIOUS HEARING CONDITION?

No. An employer generally may not ask an applicant about obvious impairments. Nor may an employer ask an applicant who has voluntarily disclosed a hearing condition any questions about its nature or severity, when it began, or how the person manages the condition. However, if an applicant has an obvious impairment or has voluntarily disclosed the existence of an impairment and the employer reasonably believes that the applicant will require an accommodation to complete the application process, or to perform the job because of the condition, the employer may ask whether the applicant will need an accommodation and what type. The employer must keep any information an applicant discloses about a medical condition confidential.

WHAT MAY AN EMPLOYER DO WHEN THEY LEARN THAT AN APPLICANT HAS OR HAD A HEARING CONDITION AFTER THE APPLICANT HAS BEEN OFFERED A JOB BUT BEFORE STARTING WORK?

When an applicant discloses, after receiving a conditional job offer, that the applicant has or had a hearing condition, an employer may ask the applicant additional questions, such as how long the individual has had the hearing condition; what, if any, hearing the applicant has; what specific hearing limitations the person experiences; and what, if any, reasonable accommodations the applicant may need to perform the job. The employer also may send the applicant for a follow-up hearing or medical examination or ask the person to submit medical documentation answering questions specifically designed to assess the applicant's ability to perform the job's functions safely. Permissible follow-up questions at this stage differ from those at the pre-offer stage, when an employer may only ask an applicant who voluntarily discloses a disability or whose disability is obvious whether the individual needs an accommodation either in the application process or to perform the job.

An employer may not withdraw an offer from an applicant with a hearing disability if the individual is able to perform the essential functions of a job, with or without reasonable accommodation, without posing a direct threat (that is, a significant risk of substantial harm) to the health or safety of the applicant or others that cannot be eliminated or reduced through reasonable accommodation.

WHEN MAY AN EMPLOYER ASK AN EMPLOYEE IF A HEARING CONDITION, OR SOME OTHER MEDICAL CONDITION, MAY BE CAUSING THE EMPLOYEE'S PERFORMANCE PROBLEMS?

Generally, an employer may ask disability-related questions or require an employee to have a medical examination when they know about a particular employee's medical condition, have observed performance problems, and reasonably believe that the problems are related to a medical condition. At other times, an employer may ask for medical information when they have observed symptoms, such as difficulties hearing, or have received reliable information from someone else (i.e., a family member or co-worker) indicating that the employee may have a medical condition that is causing performance problems. Often, however, poor job performance is unrelated to a medical condition and generally should be handled in accordance with an employer's existing policies concerning performance.

WHAT KINDS OF REASONABLE ACCOMMODATIONS ARE RELATED TO THE BENEFITS AND PRIVILEGES OF EMPLOYMENT?

Reasonable accommodations related to the benefits and privileges of employment include accommodations that are necessary to provide individuals with disabilities access to facilities or portions of facilities to which all employees are granted access (i.e., employee break rooms and cafeterias), access to information communicated in the workplace, and the opportunity to participate in employer-sponsored training and social events.

WHAT SHOULD AN EMPLOYER DO WHEN ANOTHER FEDERAL LAW PROHIBITS HIRING INDIVIDUALS WITH A HEARING CONDITION FOR PARTICULAR POSITIONS?

If a federal law prohibits an employer from hiring a person with a hearing condition for a particular position, the employer is not liable under the ADA. The employer should be certain, however, that compliance with the law actually is required, not voluntary. The employer also should be sure that the law does not contain any exceptions or waivers.

WHAT SHOULD EMPLOYERS DO TO PREVENT AND CORRECT HARASSMENT?

Employers should make clear that they will not tolerate harassment based on disability or on any other protected basis. This can be done in a number of ways, such as through a written policy, employee handbooks, staff meetings, and periodic training. The employer should emphasize that harassment is prohibited and that employees should promptly report such conduct to a manager. Finally, the employer should immediately conduct a thorough investigation of any report of harassment and take swift and appropriate corrective action.[1]

---

[1] "Hearing Disabilities in the Workplace and the Americans with Disabilities Act," U.S. Equal Employment Opportunity Commission (EEOC), January 24, 2023. Available online. URL: www.eeoc.gov/laws/guidance/hearing-disabilities-workplace-and-americans-disabilities-act. Accessed October 10, 2024.

Chapter 22 | **Support Structures for Auditory Impairment**

Chapter Contents
Section 22.1—Supports in Hotels and Motels 202
Section 22.2—Supports in Hospital Settings........................... 204

Section 22.1 | Supports in Hotels and Motels

Many people who are deaf or hard of hearing use a variety of ways to communicate. Some rely on sign language interpreters or assistive listening devices; others rely primarily on written messages. Many can speak but are not able to hear words spoken by others. The method of communication and the services or aids hotel staff must provide will vary depending on the abilities of the guest and on the complexity and nature of the communications that are required.

ADA COMPLIANCE FOR HOTELS
Under the Americans with Disabilities Act (ADA), hotels and motels must provide effective means of communication for people who are deaf or hard of hearing to ensure that they have an equal opportunity to enjoy the goods, services, accommodations, and amenities offered.

EFFECTIVE COMMUNICATION STRATEGIES
For short and relatively simple in-person conversations, such as inquiries about room rates and availability or questions about restaurant menu items, an exchange of written notes may be effective.

Many people who are deaf or hard of hearing use a teletypewriter (TTY, also known as a "TDD") rather than standard telephones for telephone communications. These devices have a keyboard and a visual display for exchanging written messages over the telephone.

PROVISION OF TTY SERVICES
To allow guests with hearing disabilities access to hotel telephone services, the hotel must provide a TTY, on request, for use in guest rooms. The hotel also will need to have a TTY at the front desk and perhaps at other telephone stations for handling billing inquiries, taking room service orders, or responding to other guest calls. Hotel desk staff should be trained in handling TTY equipment.

NATIONWIDE RELAY NETWORK
The ADA established a free nationwide relay network to handle voice-to-TTY and TTY-to-voice calls. People may use this network

to call the hotel from a TTY. The relay consists of an operator with a TTY who receives the call from a TTY user and then places the call to the hotel. The caller types the message into the TTY, and the operator relays the message by voice to the hotel staff person, listens to the staff person's response, and types the response back to the caller using the TTY. The hotel must be prepared to take and respond to relay system calls, which may take a little longer than voice calls. For outgoing calls to a TTY user, simply dial 711 to reach a relay operator.

ACCESSIBILITY FEATURES IN GUEST ROOMS

Where televisions are provided in guest rooms, closed caption decoders must be provided upon request. New televisions at least 13 inches or larger have such devices built in.

Some people with hearing disabilities use service animals—often "Hearing Ear Dogs"—to assist them with safety and way-finding. The hotel must permit guests to bring such animals into areas of the hotel where guests are normally allowed to go, even if it otherwise prohibits animals in the facility. For further information on the ADA's requirements for service animals, please see the "ADA Business Brief: Service Animals," which is available from the ADA Information Line.

If communication with guests is lengthy or complex, a sign language interpreter, an oral interpreter, or computer-assisted, real-time captioning may be necessary to ensure effective communication with people who are deaf or hard of hearing.

BUILT-IN COMMUNICATION FEATURES

Hotels and motels must also provide built-in communication features in a certain percentage of guest rooms.

These features include:
- visual alarms in guest rooms that are connected to the building's emergency alarm system
- visual notification devices in guest rooms to alert people with hearing impairments to incoming telephone calls and door knocks or bells
- electrical outlets to facilitate the use of text telephones

These communication features are required in hotel facilities built or altered after the effective date of the ADA. They are also required in hotel facilities built before the effective date of the ADA to meet the ongoing obligation to remove physical and communication barriers to the extent possible without much difficulty or expense. Hotels and motels may also use portable visual alarms and communication devices to satisfy these requirements.[1]

Section 22.2 | Supports in Hospital Settings

Many people who are deaf or hard of hearing use a variety of ways to communicate. Some rely on sign language interpreters or assistive listening devices; others rely primarily on written messages. Many can speak even though they cannot hear. The method of communication and the services or aids the hospital must provide will vary depending on the abilities of the person who is deaf or hard of hearing and on the complexity and nature of the communications that are required. Effective communication is particularly critical in health-care settings where miscommunication may lead to misdiagnosis and improper or delayed medical treatment.

ADA REQUIREMENTS FOR HOSPITALS

Under the Americans with Disabilities Act (ADA), hospitals must provide effective means of communication for patients, family members, and hospital visitors who are deaf or hard of hearing. The ADA applies to all hospital programs and services, such as emergency room care, inpatient and outpatient services, surgery, clinics, educational classes, and cafeteria and gift shop services. Wherever patients, their family members, companions, or members of the public are interacting with hospital staff, the hospital is obligated to provide effective communication.

---

[1] ADA.gov, "Communicating with Guests Who Are Deaf or Hard of Hearing in Hotels, Motels, and Other Places of Transient Lodging," U.S. Department of Justice (DOJ), August 11, 2005. Available online. URL: www.ada.gov/hotelcombr.htm. Accessed October 14, 2024.

STRATEGIES FOR EFFECTIVE COMMUNICATION

For brief and relatively simple face-to-face conversations, such as a visitor's inquiry about a patient's room number or purchase in the gift shop or cafeteria, exchanging written notes or pointing to items for purchase will likely be effective communication.

Written forms or information sheets may provide effective communication in situations where interactive communication is not necessary, such as when providing billing and insurance information or filling out admission forms and medical history inquiries.

For more complicated and interactive communications, such as a patient's discussion of symptoms with medical personnel, a physician's presentation of diagnosis and treatment options to patients or family members, or a group therapy session, a qualified sign language interpreter or other interpreters may be necessary.

TYPES OF INTERPRETERS
Sign Language Interpreters

Many people who are deaf or hard of hearing use sign language. It is a visually interactive language that uses a combination of hand motions, body gestures, and facial expressions. There are several different types of sign language, including American Sign Language (ASL) and Signed English.

Oral Interpreters

Not all people who are deaf or hard of hearing are trained in sign language. Some individuals with hearing disabilities are trained in speechreading (lipreading) and can understand spoken words fairly well with assistance from an oral interpreter. Oral interpreters are specially trained to articulate speech silently and clearly, sometimes rephrasing words or phrases to give higher visibility on the lips. Natural body language and gestures are also used.

Cued Speech Interpreters

A cued speech interpreter functions in the same manner as an oral interpreter except that he or she also uses a hand code, or cue, to represent each speech sound.

Computer Assisted Real-Time Transcription

Many people who are deaf or hard of hearing are not trained in sign language or speech reading. Computer Assisted Real-Time Transcription (CART) is a service in which an operator types what is said into a computer, which displays the typed words on a screen.

SITUATIONS WHERE AN INTERPRETER MAY BE REQUIRED FOR EFFECTIVE COMMUNICATION

- discussing a patient's symptoms and medical condition, medications, and medical history
- explaining and describing medical conditions, tests, treatment options, medications, surgery, and other procedures
- providing a diagnosis, prognosis, and recommendation for treatment
- obtaining informed consent for treatment
- communicating with a patient during treatment, testing procedures, and during physician's rounds
- providing instructions for medications, posttreatment activities, and follow-up treatments
- providing mental health services, including group or individual therapy, or counseling for patients and family members
- providing information about blood or organ donations
- explaining living wills and powers of attorney
- discussing complex billing or insurance matters
- making educational presentations, such as:
  - birthing and new parent classes
  - nutrition and weight management counseling
  - CPR (cardiopulmonary resuscitation) and first aid training

ACCOMMODATING FAMILY MEMBERS OR COMPANIONS

Hospitals may need to provide an interpreter or other assistive service in a variety of situations where it is a family member or companion rather than the patient who is deaf or hard of hearing. For example, an interpreter may be necessary to communicate where the guardian of a minor patient is deaf, to discuss prognosis and treatment options with a patient's spouse or partner who is hard of hearing, or to allow meaningful participation in a birthing class for a prospective new father who is deaf.

QUALIFICATIONS AND AVAILABILITY OF INTERPRETERS
Sign language or other interpreters must be qualified. An interpreter is qualified if he or she can interpret competently, accurately, and impartially. In the hospital setting, the interpreter must be familiar with any specialized vocabulary used and must be able to interpret medical terms and concepts. Hospital personnel who have limited familiarity with sign language should interpret only in emergency situations for a brief time until a qualified interpreter can be present.

It is inappropriate to ask family members or other companions to interpret for a person who is deaf or hard of hearing. Family members may be unable to interpret accurately in the emotional situation that often exists in a medical emergency.

Hospitals should have arrangements in place to ensure that qualified interpreters are readily available on a scheduled basis and on an unscheduled basis with minimal delay, including on-call arrangements for after-hours emergencies. Larger facilities may choose to have interpreters on staff.

Hospitals cannot charge patients or other people with hearing disabilities an extra fee for interpreter services or other communication aids and services.

TELEPHONE COMMUNICATIONS
Many people who are deaf or hard of hearing use a teletypewriter (TTY, also known as a "TDD") rather than a standard telephone. These devices have a keyboard and a visual display for exchanging written messages over the telephone.

The ADA established a free nationwide relay network to handle voice-to-TTY and TTY-to-voice calls. Individuals may use this network to call the hospital from a TTY. The relay consists of an operator with a TTY who receives the call from a TTY user and then places the call to the hospital. The caller types the message into the TTY, and the operator relays the message by voice to the hospital staff person, listens to the staff person's response, and types the response back to the caller using the TTY. The hospital must be prepared to make and receive relay system calls, which may take a little longer than voice calls. For outgoing calls to a TTY user, simply dial 711 to reach a relay operator.

ACCESSIBLE EQUIPMENT IN PATIENT ROOMS
If telephones and televisions are provided in patient rooms, the hospital must provide patients who are deaf or hard of hearing comparable accessible equipment upon request, including TTYs, telephones that are hearing aid compatible and have volume control, and televisions with closed captioning or decoders.

Visual alarms are not required in patient rooms. However, hospital evacuation procedures should include specific measures to ensure the safety of patients and visitors who are deaf or hard of hearing.

A hospital need not provide communication aids or services if doing so would fundamentally alter the nature of the goods or services offered or would result in an undue burden.

BUILT-IN COMMUNICATION FEATURES REQUIRED FOR HOSPITALS
Certain built-in communication features are required for hospitals built or altered after the effective date of the ADA:
- Visual alarms must be provided in all public and common-use areas, including restrooms, where audible alarms are provided.
- TTYs must be provided at public pay phones serving emergency, recovery, or waiting rooms, and at least one must be provided at other locations with four or more pay phones.
- A certain percentage of public phones must have other features, such as TTY plug-in capability, volume controls, and hearing aid compatibility. For more specific information, consult the ADA Standards for Accessible Design (www.ada.gov/law-and-regs/design-standards).[1]

---

[1] ADA.gov, "Communicating with People Who Are Deaf or Hard of Hearing in Hospital Settings," U.S. Department of Justice (DOJ), August 11, 2005. Available online. URL: www.ada.gov/hospcombr.htm. Accessed October 14, 2024.

Chapter 23 | Service Animals: Rights and Responsibilities

Many people with disabilities use a service animal to fully participate in everyday life. Dogs can be trained to perform various important tasks to assist individuals with disabilities, such as providing stability for a person who has difficulty walking, picking up items for a person who uses a wheelchair, preventing a child with autism from wandering away, or alerting a person with hearing loss when someone is approaching from behind.

DEFINITION OF A SERVICE ANIMAL
What Is a Service Animal?
Under the Americans with Disabilities Act (ADA), a service animal is defined as a dog that has been individually trained to do work or perform tasks for a person with a disability. The tasks performed by the dog must be directly related to the person's disability.

What Does "Do Work or Perform Tasks" Mean?
The dog must be trained to take a specific action when needed to assist the person with a disability. For example, a person with diabetes may have a dog that is trained to alert them when their blood sugar reaches high or low levels. A person with depression may have a dog that is trained to remind them to take their medication. Or, a person who has epilepsy may have a dog that is trained to detect the onset of a seizure and then help the person remain safe during the seizure.

Are "Emotional Support," "Therapy," "Comfort," or "Companion Animals" Considered Service Animals under the ADA?

No. These terms are used to describe animals that provide comfort just by being with a person. Because they have not been trained to perform a specific job or task, they do not qualify as service animals under the ADA. However, some state or local governments have laws that allow people to take emotional support animals into public places. You may check with your state and local government agencies to find out about these laws.

Does the ADA Require Service Animals to Be Professionally Trained?

No. People with disabilities have the right to train the dog themselves and are not required to use a professional service dog training program.

GENERAL RULES
Who Is Responsible for the Care and Supervision of a Service Animal?

The handler is responsible for caring for and supervising the service animal, which includes toileting, feeding, grooming, and veterinary care. Covered entities are not obligated to supervise or otherwise care for a service animal.

Can People Bring More than One Service Animal into a Public Place?

Generally, yes. Some people with disabilities may use more than one service animal to perform different tasks. For example, a person who has a visual disability and a seizure disorder may use one service animal to assist with way-finding and another that is trained as a seizure-alert dog. Other people may need two service animals for the same task, such as a person who needs two dogs to assist them with stability when walking. Staff may ask the two permissible questions about each of the dogs. If both dogs can be accommodated, both should be allowed in. In some circumstances, however, it may not be possible to accommodate more than one service animal. For example, in a crowded small restaurant, only one dog may be able to fit under the table. The only other place for the second dog would be in the aisle, which would block the space between tables. In this case, staff may request that one of the dogs be left outside.

CERTIFICATION AND REGISTRATION
Does the ADA Require That Service Animals Be Certified as Service Animals?
No. Covered entities may not require documentation, such as proof that the animal has been certified, trained, or licensed as a service animal, as a condition for entry.

My City Requires All Dogs to Be Registered and Licensed. Does This Apply to My Service Animal?
Yes. Service animals are subject to local dog licensing and registration requirements.

My City Requires All Dogs to Be Vaccinated. Does This Apply to My Service Animal?
Yes. Individuals who have service animals are not exempt from local animal control or public health requirements.

BREEDS
Can Service Animals Be Any Breed of Dog?
Yes. The ADA does not restrict the type of dog breeds that can be service animals.

Can Individuals with Disabilities Be Refused Access to a Facility Based Solely on the Breed of Their Service Animal?
No. A service animal may not be excluded based on assumptions or stereotypes about the animal's breed or how the animal might behave. However, if a particular service animal behaves in a way that poses a direct threat to the health or safety of others, has a history of such behavior, or is not under the control of the handler, that animal may be excluded. If an animal is excluded for such reasons, staff must still offer their goods or services to the person without the animal present.

EXCLUSION OF SERVICE ANIMALS
When Can Service Animals Be Excluded?
The ADA does not require covered entities to modify policies, practices, or procedures if it would "fundamentally alter" the nature of the goods, services, programs, or activities provided to the public. Nor does it overrule legitimate safety requirements. If admitting service animals would fundamentally alter the nature of a service or program, service animals may be prohibited. In addition, if a particular service animal is out of control and the handler does not take effective action to control it, or if it is not housebroken, that animal may be excluded.

MISCELLANEOUS
Are Stores Required to Allow Service Animals to Be Placed in a Shopping Cart?
Generally, the dog must stay on the floor, or the person must carry the dog. For example, if a person with diabetes has a glucose-alert dog, they may carry the dog in a chest pack so it can be close to their face, allowing the dog to smell their breath and alert them of a change in glucose levels.

Are Churches, Temples, Synagogues, Mosques, and Other Places of Worship Required to Allow Individuals to Bring Their Service Animals into the Facility?
No. Religious institutions and organizations are specifically exempt from the ADA requirements. However, certain state laws may apply to religious organizations.

Do Federal Agencies, Such as the U.S. Department of Veterans Affairs, Have to Comply with the ADA?
No. Section 504 of the Rehabilitation Act of 1973 is the federal law that protects the rights of people with disabilities to participate in federal programs and services. For information or to file a complaint, contact the agency's equal opportunity office.

Do Commercial Airlines Have to Comply with the ADA?

No. The Air Carrier Access Act is a federal law that protects the rights of people with disabilities in air travel. For information or to file a complaint, contact the U.S. Department of Transportation, Aviation Consumer Protection Division (www.transportation.gov/airconsumer), at 202-366-2220.[1]

---

[1] ADA.gov, "Frequently Asked Questions about Service Animals and the ADA," U.S. Department of Justice (DOJ), February 28, 2020. Available online. URL: www.ada.gov/regs2010/service_animal_qa.html. Accessed October 14, 2024.

Chapter 24 | Education

Chapter Contents
Section 24.1—Federal Requirements for Communication Access
　　　　　in Education..216
Section 24.2—Testing Accommodations and Disability Rights.............218

Section 24.1 | Federal Requirements for Communication Access in Education

WHAT DO FEDERAL LAWS REQUIRE OF A PUBLIC SCHOOL TO MEET THE COMMUNICATION NEEDS OF STUDENTS WITH HEARING OR SPEECH DISABILITIES?

Under the Individuals with Disabilities Education Act (IDEA), schools must provide a student with a disability a free appropriate public education (FAPE) designed to provide meaningful educational benefit through an Individualized Education Program (IEP).

Under Title II of the Americans with Disabilities Act (ADA), schools must, without charge, ensure that communication with students with disabilities is as effective as communication with students without disabilities, giving primary consideration to students and parents in determining which auxiliary aids and services are necessary to provide such effective communication.

WILL THE AIDS AND SERVICES REQUIRED BE THE SAME UNDER BOTH FEDERAL LAWS?

It depends on the individual needs of the particular student.

Sometimes the special education and related services provided to a student as part of FAPE under the IDEA will also meet the Title II requirements. In other instances, in order to meet the Title II requirements, a school might have to provide a student with aids or services that are not required by FAPE.

Some services related to communication, such as teaching a child to understand sign language, are not required by Title II's effective communication requirement but may be required by FAPE.

DOES THE SCHOOL HAVE TO GIVE A STUDENT THE AID OR SERVICE THE PARENTS REQUEST?

Under Title II, the school must provide the aid or service requested unless the school can prove that a different auxiliary aid or service is as effective in meeting the student's communication needs (in which case the school must provide that alternative), or the school can prove that the aid or service would result in a fundamental alteration or in undue financial and administrative burdens (in which case the school must take other steps to ensure that the student can participate).

Schools are not required to provide more aids or services than what is needed to ensure effective communication or to comply with requests about details of the aid or service (such as particular brands or models) that are not relevant to its effectiveness.

WHAT TYPES OF AIDS OR SERVICES COULD BE REQUIRED FOR STUDENTS?

There are no categorical rules. A school must assess the needs of each individual.

For a student who is deaf, deaf-blind, or hard of hearing, some examples are the exchange of written materials, interpreters, note takers, real-time computer-aided transcription services (e.g., CART), assistive listening systems, accessible electronic and information technology, and open and closed captioning.

For a student with a speech disability, some examples are a word or letter board, writing materials, spelling to communicate, a qualified sign language interpreter, a portable device that writes and/or produces speech, and telecommunications services.

WHERE CAN I GET MORE INFORMATION ABOUT THE RIGHTS OF STUDENTS WITH HEARING OR SPEECH DISABILITIES?

The U.S. Department of Education's Office for Civil Rights (OCR) and Office of Special Education and Rehabilitative Services, along with the U.S. Department of Justice (DOJ), have issued a Dear Colleague Letter and a Frequently Asked Questions document explaining what federal law requires of schools to meet the communication needs of students with hearing or speech disabilities.

WHAT CAN A PARENT DO IF THE SCHOOL WILL NOT GIVE A CHILD WHAT THE PARENT THINKS IS NEEDED?

Arrange to meet with the IEP or 504 team or the school's Title II or 504 Coordinator. Consider using the school district's published disability grievance procedures.

Under the IDEA, a parent challenging the provision of FAPE may request mediation, file a complaint with the state educational agency, or file a due process complaint to request an impartial administrative hearing.

Under Title II, a parent may choose to file a lawsuit in court. Parents of an IDEA-eligible student generally must exhaust the administrative hearing procedures of the IDEA, which means obtaining a final decision under the IDEA's impartial due process hearing procedures, before filing a lawsuit seeking a remedy that is also available under the IDEA.[1]

Section 24.2 | Testing Accommodations and Disability Rights

Standardized examinations and other high-stakes tests are gateways to educational and employment opportunities. Whether seeking admission to a high school, college, or graduate program, or attempting to obtain a professional license or certification for a trade, it is difficult to achieve such goals without sitting for some kind of standardized exam or high-stakes test. While many testing entities have made efforts to ensure equal opportunity for individuals with disabilities, the Department continues to receive questions and complaints relating to excessive and burdensome documentation demands, failures to provide needed testing accommodations, and failures to respond to requests for testing accommodations in a timely manner.

The Americans with Disabilities Act (ADA) ensures that individuals with disabilities have the opportunity to fairly compete for and pursue such opportunities by requiring testing entities to offer exams in a manner that is accessible to people with disabilities.

---

[1] ADA.gov, "Meeting the Communication Needs of Students with Hearing, Vision, or Speech Disabilities," U.S. Department of Justice (DOJ), November 12, 2014. Available online. URL: www.ada.gov/doe_doj_eff_comm/doe_doj_eff_comm_fact_sht.htm. Accessed October 12, 2024.

When needed testing accommodations are provided, test-takers can demonstrate their true aptitude.

WHAT ARE TESTING ACCOMMODATIONS?
Testing accommodations are changes to the regular testing environment and auxiliary aids and services that allow individuals with disabilities to demonstrate their true aptitude or achievement level on standardized exams or other high-stakes tests.

Examples of the wide range of testing accommodations that may be required include:
- Braille or large-print exam booklets
- screen reading technology
- scribes to transfer answers to Scantron bubble sheets or record dictated notes and essays
- extended time
- wheelchair-accessible testing stations
- distraction-free rooms
- physical prompts (such as for individuals with hearing impairments)
- permission to bring and take medications during the exam (i.e., for individuals with diabetes who must monitor their blood sugar and administer insulin)

WHAT KINDS OF TESTS ARE COVERED?
Exams administered by any private, state, or local government entity related to applications, licensing, certification, or credentialing for secondary or postsecondary education, professional, or trade purposes are covered by the ADA, and testing accommodations must be provided pursuant to the ADA.

Examples of covered exams include:
- high school equivalency exams (such as the GED)
- high school entrance exams (such as the SSAT or ISEE)
- college entrance exams (such as the SAT or ACT)
- exams for admission to professional schools (such as the LSAT or MCAT)
- admissions exams for graduate schools (such as the GRE or GMAT)

- licensing exams for trade purposes (such as cosmetology) or professional purposes (such as bar exams or medical licensing exams, including clinical assessments)

WHO IS ELIGIBLE TO RECEIVE TESTING ACCOMMODATIONS?

- **Individuals with disabilities are eligible to receive necessary testing accommodations.** Under the ADA, an individual with a disability is a person who has a physical or mental impairment that substantially limits a major life activity (such as seeing, hearing, learning, reading, concentrating, or thinking) or a major bodily function (such as the neurological, endocrine, or digestive system). The determination of whether an individual has a disability generally should not demand extensive analysis and must be made without regard to any positive effects of measures such as medication, medical supplies or equipment, low-vision devices (other than ordinary eyeglasses or contact lenses), prosthetics, hearing aids and cochlear implants, or mobility devices. However, negative effects, such as side effects of medication or burdens associated with following a particular treatment regimen, may be considered when determining whether an individual's impairment substantially limits a major life activity.
- **A substantial limitation of a major life activity may be based on the extent to which the impairment affects the condition, manner, or duration in which the individual performs the major life activity.** To be "substantially limited" in a major life activity does not require that the person be unable to perform the activity. In determining whether an individual is substantially limited in a major life activity, it may be useful to consider, when compared to most people in the general population, the conditions under which the individual performs the activity or the manner in which the activity is performed. It may also be useful to consider the length of time an individual can perform a major life activity or the length of time it takes an individual to perform a major life activity, as compared to most people in the general population.

- **A person with a history of academic success may still be a person with a disability who is entitled to testing accommodations under the ADA.** A history of academic success does not mean that a person does not have a disability that requires testing accommodations. For example, someone with a learning disability may achieve a high level of academic success but may nevertheless be substantially limited in one or more of the major life activities of reading, writing, speaking, or learning, because of the additional time or effort he or she must spend to read, write, speak, or learn compared to most people in the general population.

WHAT TESTING ACCOMMODATIONS MUST BE PROVIDED?

Testing entities must ensure that the test scores of individuals with disabilities accurately reflect the individual's aptitude or achievement level or whatever skill the exam or test is intended to measure. A testing entity must administer its exam so that it accurately reflects an individual's aptitude, achievement level, or skill that the exam purports to measure rather than the individual's impairment (except where the impaired skill is one the exam purports to measure).

WHAT KIND OF DOCUMENTATION IS SUFFICIENT TO SUPPORT A REQUEST FOR TESTING ACCOMMODATIONS?

All testing entities must adhere to the following principles regarding what may and may not be required when a person with a disability requests testing accommodation.

- **Documentation**. Any documentation required by a testing entity in support of a request for testing accommodations must be reasonable and limited to the need for the requested testing accommodations.
- **Past testing accommodations**. Proof of past testing accommodations in similar test settings is generally sufficient to support a request for the same testing accommodations for a current standardized exam or other high-stakes test.
- **Formal public school accommodations**. If a candidate previously received testing accommodations under an

Individualized Education Program (IEP) or a Section 504 Plan, he or she should generally receive the same testing accommodations for a current standardized exam or high-stakes test.
- **Private school testing accommodations.** If a candidate received testing accommodations in a private school for similar tests under a formal policy, he or she should generally receive the same testing accommodations for a current standardized exam or high-stakes test.
- **First-time requests or informal classroom testing accommodations.** An absence of previous formal testing accommodations does not preclude a candidate from receiving testing accommodations.
- **Qualified professionals.** Testing entities should defer to documentation from a qualified professional who has made an individualized assessment of the candidate that supports the need for the requested testing accommodations.

HOW QUICKLY SHOULD A TESTING ENTITY RESPOND TO A REQUEST FOR TESTING ACCOMMODATIONS?

A testing entity must respond in a timely manner to requests for testing accommodations to ensure equal opportunity for individuals with disabilities. Testing entities should ensure that their process for reviewing and approving testing accommodations responds in time for applicants to register and prepare for the test. In addition, the process should provide applicants with a reasonable opportunity to respond to any requests for additional information from the testing entity and still be able to take the test in the same testing cycle. Failure by a testing entity to act in a timely manner, coupled with seeking unnecessary documentation, could result in such an extended delay that it constitutes a denial of equal opportunity or equal treatment in an examination setting for people with disabilities.[1]

---

[1] ADA.gov, "Testing Accommodations," U.S. Department of Justice (DOJ), September 15, 2010. Available online. URL: www.ada.gov/regs2014/testing_accommodations.html. Accessed October 12, 2024.

Part 7 | Additional Resources

Chapter 25 | Directory of Organizations Providing Support for People with Auditory Impairment

Administration for Community Living (ACL)
330 C St., S.W.
Washington, DC 20201
Toll-Free: 800-677-1116
Phone: 202-401-4634
Website: https://acl.gov
Email: aclinfo@acl.hhs.gov

Agency for Healthcare Research and Quality (AHRQ)
5600 Fishers Ln.
7th Fl.
Rockville, MD 20857
Phone: 301-427-1364
Website: www.ahrq.gov

Centers for Disease Control and Prevention (CDC)
1600 Clifton Rd.
Atlanta, GA 30329-4027
Toll-Free: 800-CDC-INFO (800-232-4636)
Toll-Free TTY: 888-232-6348
Website: www.cdc.gov

Resources in this chapter were compiled from several sources deemed reliable; all contact information was verified and updated in November 2024.

Centers for Medicare and Medicaid Services (CMS)
7500 Security Blvd.
Baltimore, MD 21244-1850
Toll-Free: 877-267-2323
Phone: 410-786-3000
Toll-Free TTY: 866-226-1819
TTY: 410-786-0727
Website: www.cms.gov

Early Childhood Learning and Knowledge Center (ECLKC)
Toll-Free: 866-763-6481
Website: https://eclkc.ohs.acf.hhs.gov
Email: HeadStart@eclkc.info

Federal Communications Commission (FCC)
45 L St., N.E.
Washington, DC 20554
Toll-Free: 888-CALL-FCC (888-225-5322)
Phone: 202-418-1122
Toll-Free Fax: 866-418-0232
Website: www.fcc.gov

Genetic and Rare Diseases Information Center (GARD)
P.O. Box 8126
Gaithersburg, MD 20898-8126
Toll-Free: 888-205-2311
Phone: 301-251-4925
Toll-Free TTY: 888-205-3223
Fax: 301-251-4911
Website: https://rarediseases.info.nih.gov

MedlinePlus
8600 Rockville Pike
Bethesda, MD 20894
Toll-Free: 888-FIND-NLM (888-346-3656)
Phone: 301-594-5983
Website: https://medlineplus.gov

National Cancer Institute (NCI)
Toll-Free: 800-4-CANCER (800-422-6237)
Website: www.cancer.gov
Email: NCIinfo@nih.gov

National Institute of Arthritis and Musculoskeletal and Skin Diseases (NIAMS)
31 Center Dr., MSC 2350
Bldg. 31, Rm. 4C02
Bethesda, MD 20892-2350
Toll-Free: 877-22-NIAMS (877-226-4267)
Phone: 301-495-4484
Fax: 301-718-6366
Website: www.niams.nih.gov
Email: NIAMSinfo@mail.nih.gov

National Institute of Diabetes and Digestive and Kidney Diseases (NIDDK)
9000 Rockville Pike
Bethesda, MD 20892
Toll-Free: 800-860-8747
Website: www.niddk.nih.gov
Email: healthinfo@niddk.nih.gov

National Institute of Neurological Disorders and Stroke (NINDS)
P.O. Box 5801
Bethesda, MD 20824
Toll-Free: 800-352-9424
Website: www.ninds.nih.gov

National Institute on Aging (NIA)
31 Center Dr.
Bldg. 31, Rm. 5C27
Bethesda, MD 20892
Toll-Free: 800-222-2225
Website: www.nia.nih.gov
Email: niaic@nia.nih.gov

National Institute on Deafness and Other Communication Disorders (NIDCD)
1 Communication Ave.
Bethesda, MD 20892-3456
Toll-Free Phone: 800-241-1044
Toll-Free TTY: 800-241-1055
Website: www.nidcd.nih.gov
Email: nidcdinfo@nidcd.nih.gov

National Institute on Drug Abuse (NIDA)
16071 Industrial Dr., Dock 11
Phone: 301-443-6441
Website: https://nida.nih.gov

National Institutes of Health (NIH)
9000 Rockville Pike
Bethesda, MD 20892
Phone: 301-496-4000
TTY: 301-402-9612
Website: www.nih.gov

Occupational Safety and Health Administration (OSHA)
200 Constitution Ave., N.W.
Rm. N3626
Washington, DC 20210
Toll-Free: 800-321-OSHA (800-321-6742)
Website: www.osha.gov

Office of Disease Prevention and Health Promotion (ODPHP)
1101 Wootton Pkwy., Ste. 420
Rockville, MD 20852
Website: https://health.gov

U.S. Department of Education (ED)
400 Maryland Ave., S.W.
Washington, DC 20202
Toll-Free: 800-USA-LEARN (800-872-5327)
Phone: 202-401-2000
Website: www.ed.gov
Email: ocr@ed.gov

U.S. Department of Health and Human Services (HHS)
200 Independence Ave., S.W.
Washington, DC 20201
Toll-Free: 877-696-6775
Website: www.hhs.gov

U.S. Department of Justice (DOJ)
950 Pennsylvania Ave., N.W.
Washington, DC 20530-0001
Phone: 202-514-2000
Toll-Free TTY/TDD: 800-877-8339
Website: www.justice.gov

U.S. Department of Veterans Affairs (VA)
Toll-Free: 800-698-2411
Toll-Free TTY: 800-698-2711
Website: www.va.gov

U.S. Environmental Protection Agency (EPA)
1200 Pennsylvania Ave., N.W.
Washington, DC 20460
Phone: 202-564-4700
Website: www.epa.gov

U.S. Equal Employment Opportunity Commission (EEOC)
131 M St., N.E.
Washington, DC 20507
Toll-Free: 800-669-4000
Phone: 202-921-2539
Toll-Free TTY: 800-669-6820
Website: www.eeoc.gov
Email: info@eeoc.gov

U.S. Food and Drug Administration (FDA)
10903 New Hampshire Ave.
Silver Spring, MD 20993-0002
Toll-Free: 888-INFO-FDA (888-463-6332)
Website: www.fda.gov

INDEX

INDEX

INDEX

Page numbers followed by "n" refer to citation information; by "t" indicate tables; and by "f" indicate figures.

A

AABR *see* Automated Auditory Brainstem Response
AAC devices *see* augmentative and alternative communication devices
acoustic reflex, auditory system 5
acute otitis media (AOM), defined 64
ADA *see* Americans with Disabilities Act
ADA.gov
   publications
      communicating in lodging 204n
      communicating in hospital settings 208n
      communication needs of students with disabilities 218n
      disability rights laws 194n
      FAQs about service animals and the ADA 213n
      testing accommodations 222n
Administration for Community Living (ACL), contact information 225
Agency for Healthcare Research and Quality (AHRQ), contact information 225
age-related hearing loss
   auditory neuropathy 104
   described 17
   overview 115–118
ALDs *see* assistive listening devices

alerting devices
   assistive listening devices (ALDs) 179
   defined 175
American Sign Language (ASL)
   communication barriers 27
   defined 36
   sign language interpreters 205
   Video Relay Service (VRS) 41
Americans with Disabilities Act (ADA)
   defined 31
   described 189
   employment rights 195
   hearing impairments 183
   service animal 209
   sign language interpreters 202
   speech disabilities 216
amplification
   hearing aids 161
   tinnitus 94
analog aids, hearing aids 164
AOM *see* acute otitis media
ASL *see* American Sign Language
assistive devices
   hearing aids 20, 150
   hearing loss 19, 30, 86
   otoacoustic emissions test 134
   overview 175–179
assistive listening devices (ALDs)
   assistive devices 176
   auxiliary aids 32
   defined 118
assistive technology
   assistive devices 175
   described 149

233

audiogram
  hearing tests 130
  otosclerosis 97
audiography, hearing tests 130
audiologic test, hearing tests 130
audiologist
  balance disorder 101
  cochlear implant 153, 173
  hearing aids 164
  hearing loss 19, 142
  hearing problem 117
  hearing screening 128
  hearing test 132
  otosclerosis 97
  tinnitus 93
audiometry
  hearing tests 130
  sudden deafness 108
audiometry test, described 132
auditory cortex, tinnitus 93
auditory nerve
  auditory neuropathy 103
  auditory system 6
  cochlear implant 171
  depicted 5f
  gene therapy 156
  hearing loss 17, 45
  hearing tests 131
  sudden deafness 107
auditory neuropathy, overview 103–106
auditory pathway, hearing loss 10
auditory system
  auditory neuropathy 103
  hearing loss 11
  human auditory range 4
augmentative and alternative communication (AAC) devices, defined 175
auricle
  auditory system 7
  human auditory range 5
Automated Auditory Brainstem Response (AABR), hearing screening 128

B

background noise
  assistive devices 150
  hearing aids 166
  hearing loss 20, 118
  assistive listening devices (ALDs) 176
bacterial meningitis, described 68
balance disorder, overview 97–102
barriers to accessibility 26
behind-the-ear (BTE) hearing aid, depicted 163f
benign paroxysmal positional vertigo (BPPV), described 100
bilateral hearing loss 12
bone conduction, audiometry tests 133
bone-anchored hearing aids, defined 150
BPPV *see* benign paroxysmal positional vertigo
brain tumors
  hearing problems 110
  tinnitus 92
British Sign Language (BSL) 36
BSL *see* British Sign Language
BTE hearing aid *see* behind-the-ear hearing aid

C

canal aids, described 164
canal caps, defined 139
canal collapse, auditory system 7
captioned telephone
  assistive listening devices (ALDs) 179
  described 183
  Telecommunications Relay Service (TRS) 40
captioning
  auxiliary aids 32
  communication barriers 27
  defined 150
  overview 181–185
  Telecommunications Relay Service (TRS) 191

Index

CART *see* Computer Assisted Real-Time Transcription
Centers for Disease Control and Prevention (CDC)
    contact information 225
    publications
        audiometry procedures 7n, 12n
        congenital CMV and hearing loss 82n
        congenital Zika syndrome 113n
        cytomegalovirus 80n
        genetics and hearing loss 123n
        hearing loss and quality of life 25n
        hearing loss in children 15n
        intervention options 153n
        newborn hearing screening 129n
        noise-induced hearing loss 137n
        promoting hearing health in schools 143n
        treatment and intervention for hearing loss 151n
Centers for Medicare and Medicaid Services (CMS), contact information 226
cerumen, auditory system 7
chronic otitis media with effusion, defined 64
CIC hearing aid *see* completely-in-canal hearing aid
CMV *see* cytomegalovirus
cochlea
    auditory brainstem implants 150
    balance disorders 99
    depicted 5f, 83f
    gene therapy 156
    hearing loss 10, 121
    hearing tests 130
    human auditory range 6
    vestibular aqueducts 82
cochlear implant
    assistive listening devices (ALDs) 177
    auditory brainstem implants 149
    auditory neuropathy 105
    defined 118
    described 20
    gene therapy 156
    hearing impairments 196
    hearing loss 15, 81
    overview 171–173
communication access, hearing impairments 182
communication barriers, described 27
communication disorders
    assistive devices 175
    gene therapy 155
    hearing loss 30
completely-in-canal (CIC) hearing aid, depicted 163f
Computer Assisted Real-Time Transcription (CART)
    defined 206
    speech disabilities 217
conductive hearing loss
    hearing loss 152
    hearing tests 130
    otoacoustic emissions test 134
    sudden deafness 108
congenital Zika virus, congenital Zika syndrome 112
cued speech
    hearing loss 86
    oral interpreters 205
cytomegalovirus (CMV) 80

D

decibel
    auditory system 3
    hearing loss 45
    hearing protectors 138
    sudden deafness 108
    workplace noise 50
digital aids, hearing aids 164
disability rights 218
dizziness
    balance disorders 98
    gene therapy 156

dizziness, *continued*
  hearing aids 169
  hearing loss 96
  Ménière disease 88
  sudden deafness 107

E

ear canal
  auditory function 7
  auditory neuropathy 105
  depicted 5f
  ear infection 66
  gene therapy 155
  hearing aids 162
  hearing loss 10
  hearing problems 111
  hearing protectors 138
  human auditory range 5
  tinnitus 17, 92
ear infection
  audiologist 129
  balance disorders 98
  children 64
  conductive hearing loss 152
  intratympanic steroid treatment 154
  perilymph fistula 101
  tinnitus 92
eardrum, depicted 5f
Early Childhood Learning and Knowledge Center (ECLKC), contact information 226
earmuffs, defined 139
earplugs, described 138
earwax *see* cerumen
edited captions, described 182
electronic newsroom captions (ENR), described 182
endolymphatic duct, depicted 83f
endolymphatic sac, depicted 83f
enlarged vestibular aqueduct
  depicted 83f
  overview 84–86
enlarged endolymphatic sac, depicted 83f

Eustachian tube
  depicted 5f
  ear infections 65
external auditory meatus *see* ear canal

F

Fair Housing Act 191
Federal Communications Commission (FCC)
  contact information 226
  publication
    Telecommunications Relay Service (TRS) 41n
fungal meningitis, described 70

G

gene therapy, overview 155–157
Genetic and Rare Diseases Information Center (GARD), contact information 226

H

hearing aids
  assistive technology 149
  auditory neuropathy 105
  auxiliary aids and services 32
  baby 129
  children 81, 148
  described 20
  hearing loss 117
  hearing test 132
  otosclerosis 97
  overview 161–166
  testing accommodations 220
  tinnitus 94
  see also over-the-counter (OTC) hearing aids
hearing impairment, employment rights 195
hearing loop 176
hearing loss
  auditory neuropathy 103
  bacterial meningitis 68

hearing loss, *continued*
   captions 181
   children 148
   communication needs 30
   cytomegalovirus (CMV) 80
   daily life 24
   enlarged vestibular aqueducts 82
   gene therapy 155
   genetic factors 119
   hearing tests 130
   late effects of cancer
      treatment 110
   noise-induced
      damage 136
   otosclerosis 96
   overview 10–21
   service animals 209
   shingles 74
   tinnitus 92
   see also age-related hearing loss;
      assistive devices; hearing aids;
      noise-induced hearing loss;
      over-the-counter (OTC)
      hearing aids
hearing protection
   overview 138–140
   schools 144
hearing screening
   baby 128
   children 14
   Ménière disease 88
   students 141
hearing test, adults 130
hearing threshold 11
herpes zoster *see* shingles

I

IDEA *see* Individuals with Disabilities
   Education Act
IEP *see* Individualized Education
   Program
incus, depicted 5f
Individualized Education Program
   (IEP) 216, 222
Individuals with Disabilities Education
   Act (IDEA) 192, 216
inner ear, depicted 5f, 83f
in-the-canal (ITC) hearing aid,
   depicted 163f
in-the-ear (ITE) hearing aid,
   depicted 163f
intratympanic steroid treatment,
   described 154
ITC hearing aid *see* in-the-canal
   hearing aid
ITE hearing aid *see* in-the-ear
   hearing aid

L

labyrinthitis, described 100
lipreading
   auditory neuropathy 106
   cochlear implants 172
   oral interpreters 205
listening fatigue 24

M

Mal de Débarquement syndrome
   (MdDS), described 101
malleus, depicted 5f
MdDS *see* Mal de Débarquement
   syndrome
MedlinePlus
   contact information 226
   publication
      hearing tests for
         adults 134n
Ménière disease
   balance disorder 100
   overview 88–90
   sudden deafness 107
   tinnitus 92
meningitis, overview 67–73
middle ear, depicted 5f
mini behind-the-ear (BTE) hearing
   aid, depicted 163f
mixed hearing loss,
   defined 131

N

National Cancer Institute (NCI)
  contact information 227
  publication
    childhood cancer treatment and late effects 111n
National Center on Birth Defects and Developmental Disabilities (NCBDDD)
  publication
    disability barriers to inclusion 29n
National Institute for Occupational Safety and Health (NIOSH)
  publications
    aircrew and noise 53n
    engineering controls 59n
    hearing disorders risk reduction for musicians 52n
    hearing loss in forestry and logging 56n
    hearing protection 140n
National Institute of Arthritis and Musculoskeletal and Skin Diseases (NIAMS), contact information 227
National Institute of Diabetes and Digestive and Kidney Diseases (NIDDK), contact information 227
National Institute of Neurological Disorders and Stroke (NINDS)
  contact information 227
  publication
    meningitis 73n
National Institute on Aging (NIA)
  contact information 227
  publications
    hearing loss in older adults 21n
    shingles 77n
National Institute on Deafness and Other Communication Disorders (NIDCD)
  contact information 228
  publications
    age-related hearing loss (presbycusis) 118n
    American Sign Language (ASL) 38n
    assistive devices 179n
    auditory neuropathy 106n
    balance disorders 102n
    captions for deaf and hard of hearing viewers 185n
    children and noise-induced hearing loss 146n
    cochlear implants 173n
    communication 31n
    ear infections in children 67n
    enlarged vestibular aqueducts and childhood hearing loss 86n
    hearing aids 166n
    Ménière's disease 90n
    noise-induced hearing loss 47n
    otosclerosis 97n
    over-the-counter (OTC) hearing aids 170n
    sudden deafness 109n
    tinnitus 95n
National Institute on Drug Abuse (NIDA), contact information 228
National Institutes of Health (NIH)
  contact information 228
  publications
    gene therapy for hearing loss 157n
    steroid treatments for sudden deafness 155n
neonatal intensive care unit (NICU) 14
nerve deafness *see* sensorineural hearing loss
NICU *see* neonatal intensive care unit
noise control, hearing health 51
noise exposure
  hearing health 50
  hearing protectors 138
  tinnitus 91

noise-induced hearing loss
    exposure levels 53
    hearing health 50
    overview 45–47
    prevention 137
    schools 140, 144

O

occupational hearing loss
    aviation 52
    forestry 54
Occupational Safety and Health
    Administration (OSHA)
    contact information 228
    publication
        occupational noise
            exposure 51n
Office of Disease Prevention and
    Health Promotion (ODPHP),
    contact information 228
OM *see* otitis media
OME *see* otitis media with effusion
open and closed captions,
    described 182
oral interpreter
    guest rooms 203
    hospitals 205
otitis media (OM), described 64
otitis media with effusion (OME),
    described 64
otoacoustic emissions test,
    described 134
otolaryngologist
    age-related hearing loss 117
    auditory neuropathy 104
    balance disorder 102
    bone conduction test 133
    enlarged vestibular aqueducts 85
    hearing test 132
    otosclerosis 97
    prescription hearing aids 167
    sudden deafness 108
    surgery 152
    tinnitus 93

otosclerosis, overview 96–97
otoscopic exam, defined 111
outer ear, depicted 5f
over-the-counter (OTC) hearing aids,
    overview 167–170

P

pediatric audiologist 129
Pendred syndrome, described 84
perilymph fistula, described 101
personal protective equipment (PPE),
    exposure to noise 56, 138
personal sound amplification products
    (PSAPs), described 168
physical barriers, described 28
pinna
    depicted 5f
    see also auricle
PPE *see* personal protective equipment
presbycusis *see* age-related hearing loss
PSAPs *see* personal sound
    amplification products
pure tone audiometry, sudden
    deafness 108

Q

qualified interpreter
    auxiliary aids and services 32
    hospitals 207

R

real-time captioning
    described 182
    guest rooms 203
rear-window captioning, described 183
relay services *see* Telecommunications
    Relay Service

S

semicircular canals, depicted 5f
sensorineural hearing loss
    children 84
    defined 10
    hearing aids 161

service animal
    guest rooms 203
    overview 209–213
shingles, overview 73–77
sign language
    adults 172
    auditory neuropathy 106
    children 81, 148
    interpreters 205
SLP *see* speech-language pathologist
sound amplification, tinnitus 94
sound test 130
speech discrimination test 132
speech perception, auditory
    neuropathy 103
speech-language pathologist (SLP)
    cochlear implant 153
    hearing loss prevention 142
speechreading, interpreters 205
stapes, depicted 5f
sudden deafness
    overview 106–109
    steroid treatments 153
sudden sensorineural hearing loss *see*
    sudden deafness
surgery
    children 152
    cochlear device 153
    conductive hearing loss 131
    Ménière disease 90
    otosclerosis 97
    perilymph fistula 101

T

Telecommunications Act of 1996,
    defined 183
Telecommunications Relay Service (TRS)
    ADA Title IV 191
    overview 38–41
Television Decoder Circuitry
    Act of 1990, described 183
temporal bone
    aqueducts 82
    depicted 5f
    inner ear 6

testing accommodations,
    overview 218–222
tinnitus
    hearing loss 17, 46
    hearing screening program 142
    hearing test 131
    medical attention 169
    Ménière disease 89
    mental health 25
    noise-induced hearing loss 137
    otosclerosis 96
    overview 90–95
    sudden deafness 107
TRS *see* Telecommunications Relay
    Service
tympanic membrane 7
tympanometry test,
    described 133

U

U.S. Department of Education (ED),
    contact information 228
U.S. Department of Health and
    Human Services (HHS)
    contact information 229
    publication
        effective communication 34n
U.S. Department of Justice (DOJ),
    contact information 229
U.S. Department of Veterans Affairs
    (VA), contact information 229
U.S. Environmental Protection
    Agency (EPA), contact
    information 229
U.S. Equal Employment Opportunity
    Commission (EEOC)
    contact information 229
    publication
        hearing disabilities and the
            ADA 200n
U.S. Food and Drug Administration
    (FDA), contact information 229
unilateral hearing loss, bone-anchored
    hearing aids 150

V

valganciclovir, cytomegalovirus (CMV) 82
verbatim captions 182
vestibular aqueduct
   depicted 83f
   described 82
vestibular nerve, depicted 5f
vestibular neuronitis, defined 101
Video Relay Service (VRS) 41

viral meningitis, described 69
visual alarms
   hospitals 208
   hotels 203

W

whisper test 131

Z

Zika virus infection, pregnancy 111